600

Full Body Kettlebell & Dumbbell Workouts Book for Men and Women

600
Full Body Kettlebell & Dumbbell Workouts Book for Men and Women

With Step-by-Step Guides and Images for Strength and Fat Loss with 300 Kettlebell Workouts and 300 Dumbbell & Bodyweight Exercises

Be.Bull Publishing Group

The original purchaser of this book has permission to reproduce the pages of this book for personal use only. No other parts of this publication may be reproduced in whole or in part, shared with others, stored in a retrieval system, digitized, or transmitted in any form without written permission from the publisher.

Copyright 2024, Be.Bull Publishing Group (Aria Capri International Inc). All rights reserved.

Authors:

Be.Bull Publishing Group

Mauricio Vasquez

First Printing: October 2024

ISBN 978-1-998402-77-9 (Paperback)

ISBN 978-1-998402-78-6 (Hardcover)

<u>TIPS</u>

- Adjust the number of repetitions and the time cap for the workouts according to your capabilities, skills and physical condition
- Listen to your body and don't push yourself too hard
- If you don't have enough space where to run, you can do jumping jacks. 100-meter run is approximately equivalent to 50 jumping jacks
- Walk into the gym with a workout already selected for you
- Get motivated with a fun workout playlist
- Put your phone on airplane mode
- Start your workout with some stretches
- Log the details of each workout so you can track your progress. You can track time and number of repetitions
- Enjoy your workouts

Dear valued customer,

Your opinion matters!

By leaving a review using the QR code provided, you can help fellow readers discover and enjoy this book. Your feedback will guide others in making informed decisions and enhance their reading experience.

Thank you for contributing to our reading community!

Mauricio

Disclaimer

1. Be.Bull Publishing (Aria Capri International Inc.) strongly recommends that you consult with your physician before beginning any exercise program or workout. You should be in good physical condition and be able to participate in the exercises and workouts. We are not a licensed medical care provider and represents that we have no expertise in diagnosing, examining, or treating medical conditions of any kind, or in determining the effect of any specific exercise or workout on a medical condition.
2. You should understand that when participating in any exercise or workout, there is the possibility of physical injury. If you engage in the exercises and workouts of this book, you agree that you do so at your own risk, are voluntarily participating in these activities, assume all risk of injury to yourself, and agree to release and discharge Be.Bull Publishing (Aria Capri International Inc.) from any and all claims or causes of action, known or unknown, arising out of this book and videos.
3. The information provided through this book is not intended to be a substitute for professional medical advice, diagnosis or treatment. Never disregard professional medical advice, or delay in seeking it, because of something you have read on this book or watch in the videos. Never rely on information on this book or videos in place of seeking professional medical advice.
4. Be.Bull Publishing (Aria Capri International Inc.) is not responsible or liable for any advice, course of treatment, diagnosis or any other information, services or products that you obtain through this book or videos. You are encouraged to consult with your doctor with regard to the information contained on or through this book or videos. After reading this book or watching videos from this book, you are encouraged to review the information carefully with your professional healthcare provider.

FREE DOWNLOAD

BONUS No 1 - 1000 Full-Body Workouts

To access extra 1,000 workouts to stay motivated and avoid workout boredom with endless variety, scan this QR code:

BONUS No 2- Logging Sheets of Your Kettlebell Workout Book

To access your free e-copy of this workout book, scan this QR code:

BONUS No 3- Logging Sheets of Your Dumbbell Workout Book

To access your free e-copy of this workout book, scan this QR code:

If you want to add more variety to your workouts, scan this QR code to check these workout books!

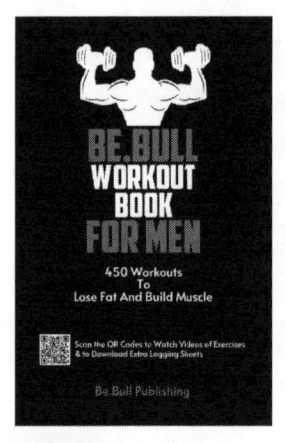

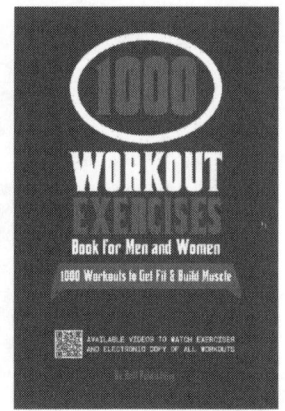

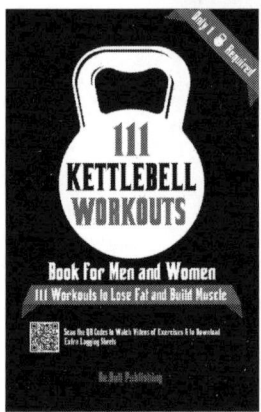

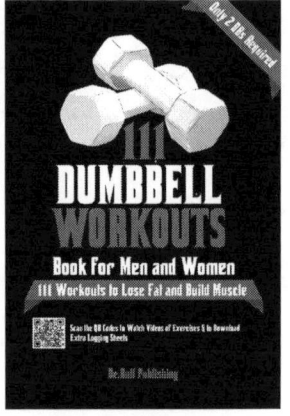

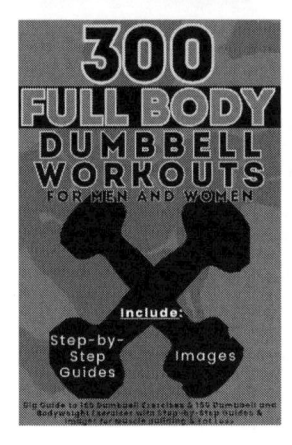

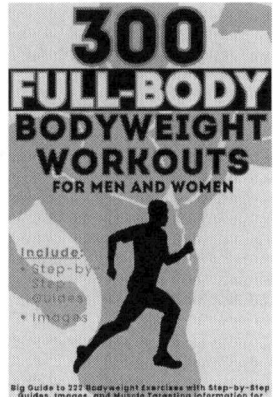

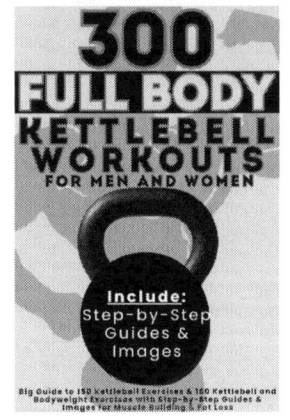

GUIDE

Part I
150 Dumbbell Only Workouts

Part II
150 Dumbbell + Body-Weight Workouts

Part III
150 Kettlebell Only Workouts

Part IV
150 Kettlebell + Body-Weight Workouts

Part I

150 Dumbbell Only Workouts

Workout No.	Workout (Dumbbell Exercises only)	Main Muscle Groups	Instructions
1	**5 Rounds for time:**		
	(1) 10 Thrusters	Shoulders, Legs, Core	Squat down, then press dumbbells overhead in one motion.
	(2) 15 Single Arm Rows (each side)	Back, Biceps, Core	Row dumbbell to hip while bent over, switch sides.
	(3) 20 Russian Twists	Core, Obliques, Shoulders	Rotate torso holding dumbbell, seated with legs lifted.
2	**As many rounds as possible in 12 mins of:**		
	(1) 10 Goblet Squats	Legs, Glutes, Core	Hold dumbbell at chest, perform deep squat.
	(2) 15 Renegade Rows	Back, Shoulders, Core	Row dumbbell from plank position, alternating sides.
	(3) 20 Hammer Curls	Biceps, Forearms	Curl dumbbells with palms facing each other.
3	**4 Rounds for time:**		
	(1) 12 Step-Ups (each leg)	Legs, Glutes, Core	Step onto platform holding dumbbells, alternating legs.
	(2) 15 Shoulder Presses	Shoulders, Triceps	Press dumbbells overhead from shoulders.
	(3) 20 V-Sit Cross Jabs	Core, Shoulders, Arms	Sit in V position, punch across body with dumbbell.
4	**Every minute on the minute for 20 mins:**		
	(1) 5 Jump Squats	Legs, Glutes, Core	Perform squat then jump, holding dumbbells.
	(2) 10 Bench Presses	Chest, Shoulders, Triceps	Press dumbbells from chest to straight arms on a bench.
	(3) 15 Russian Twists	Core, Obliques, Shoulders	Rotate torso holding dumbbell, seated with legs lifted.
5	**5 Rounds for time:**		
	(1) 10 Sumo Squats	Legs, Glutes, Core	Squat with wide stance, holding dumbbell.
	(2) 12 Seesaw Rows	Back, Biceps, Core	Row one dumbbell while other lowers, alternating.
	(3) 15 Plank Ts	Core, Shoulders, Arms	Rotate into T position from plank with dumbbell.
6	**45 secs work / 15 secs rest per exercise for 4 rounds:**		
	(1) Dumbbell Swing	Legs, Core, Shoulders	Swing dumbbell between legs then up to shoulder height.
	(2) Reverse Fly	Shoulders, Upper Back	Lift dumbbells outward while bent over.
	(3) Calf Raise	Calves, Legs	Lift heels off the ground while holding dumbbells.
7	**20 mins AMRAP (as many rounds as possible):**		
	(1) 10 Alternating Front Raises	Shoulders, Core	Lift dumbbells to shoulder height, alternating arms.
	(2) 12 Glute Bridges	Glutes, Hamstrings, Core	Lift hips while holding dumbbell on hips.
	(3) 15 Concentration Curls	Biceps	Curl dumbbell with elbow on thigh, focus on bicep.

Workout No.	Workout (Dumbbell Exercises only)	Main Muscle Groups	Instructions
8	**30 secs work / 30 secs rest per exercise for 5 rounds:**		
	(1) Farmer's Walk	Shoulders, Core, Legs	Walk holding heavy dumbbells at sides.
	(2) Reverse Lunge	Legs, Glutes, Core	Step back into lunge, holding dumbbells at sides.
	(3) Side Raise	Shoulders, Core	Lift dumbbells to sides, shoulder height.
9	**4 Rounds for time:**		
	(1) 10 Romanian Deadlifts	Hamstrings, Glutes, Lower Back	Lower dumbbells to shins with slight knee bend, then lift.
	(2) 12 Tricep Extensions	Triceps, Shoulders	Extend dumbbell overhead, bending elbow.
	(3) 15 Floor T Raises	Shoulders, Upper Back	Lift dumbbells to form T-shape while lying face down.
10	**Every minute on the minute for 16 mins:**		
	(1) 5 Goblet Squats	Legs, Glutes, Core	Hold dumbbell at chest, perform deep squat.
	(2) 10 Shoulder Presses	Shoulders, Triceps	Press dumbbells overhead from shoulders.
	(3) 15 Russian Twists	Core, Obliques, Shoulders	Rotate torso holding dumbbell, seated with legs lifted.
11	**5 Rounds for time:**		
	(1) 15 Dumbbell Pullover	Chest, Back, Core	Lower dumbbell behind head while lying on bench, then lift.
	(2) 10 Tricep Kickbacks (each arm)	Triceps, Shoulders	Extend arm backward holding dumbbell from bent-over position.
	(3) 20 Jump Squats	Legs, Glutes, Core	Perform squat then jump, holding dumbbells.
12	**As many rounds as possible in 15 mins of:**		
	(1) 12 Goblet Squats	Legs, Glutes, Core	Hold dumbbell at chest, perform deep squat.
	(2) 10 Renegade Rows	Back, Shoulders, Core	Row dumbbell from plank position, alternating sides.
	(3) 15 Russian Twists	Core, Obliques, Shoulders	Rotate torso holding dumbbell, seated with legs lifted.
13	**4 Rounds for time:**		
	(1) 10 Thrusters	Shoulders, Legs, Core	Squat down, then press dumbbells overhead in one motion.
	(2) 12 Single Arm Rows (each side)	Back, Biceps, Core	Row dumbbell to hip while bent over, switch sides.
	(3) 20 Concentration Curls	Biceps	Curl dumbbell with elbow on thigh, focus on bicep.
14	**Every minute on the minute for 18 mins:**		
	(1) 10 Bench Presses	Chest, Shoulders, Triceps	Press dumbbells from chest to straight arms on a bench.
	(2) 12 Side Raises	Shoulders, Core	Lift dumbbells to sides, shoulder height.
	(3) 15 V-Sit Cross Jabs	Core, Shoulders, Arms	Sit in V position, punch across body with dumbbell.

Workout No.	Workout (Dumbbell Exercises only)	Main Muscle Groups	Instructions
15	**5 Rounds for time:**		
	(1) 10 Sumo Squats	Legs, Glutes, Core	Squat with wide stance, holding dumbbell.
	(2) 15 Shoulder Shrugs	Shoulders, Traps	Lift shoulders toward ears holding dumbbells.
	(3) 20 Hammer Curls	Biceps, Forearms	Curl dumbbells with palms facing each other.
16	**45 secs work / 15 secs rest per exercise for 4 rounds:**		
	(1) Dumbbell Swing	Legs, Core, Shoulders	Swing dumbbell between legs then up to shoulder height.
	(2) Reverse Fly	Shoulders, Upper Back	Lift dumbbells outward while bent over.
	(3) Calf Raise	Calves, Legs	Lift heels off the ground while holding dumbbells.
17	**20 mins AMRAP (as many rounds as possible):**		
	(1) 10 Alternating Front Raises	Shoulders, Core	Lift dumbbells to shoulder height, alternating arms.
	(2) 12 Glute Bridges	Glutes, Hamstrings, Core	Lift hips while holding dumbbell on hips.
	(3) 15 Concentration Curls	Biceps	Curl dumbbell with elbow on thigh, focus on bicep.
18	**30 secs work / 30 secs rest per exercise for 5 rounds:**		
	(1) Farmer's Walk	Shoulders, Core, Legs	Walk holding heavy dumbbells at sides.
	(2) Reverse Lunge	Legs, Glutes, Core	Step back into lunge, holding dumbbells at sides.
	(3) Side Raise	Shoulders, Core	Lift dumbbells to sides, shoulder height.
19	**4 Rounds for time:**		
	(1) 10 Romanian Deadlifts	Hamstrings, Glutes, Lower Back	Lower dumbbells to shins with slight knee bend, then lift.
	(2) 12 Tricep Extensions	Triceps, Shoulders	Extend dumbbell overhead, bending elbow.
	(3) 15 Floor T Raises	Shoulders, Upper Back	Lift dumbbells to form T-shape while lying face down.
20	**Every minute on the minute for 16 mins:**		
	(1) 5 Goblet Squats	Legs, Glutes, Core	Hold dumbbell at chest, perform deep squat.
	(2) 10 Shoulder Presses	Shoulders, Triceps	Press dumbbells overhead from shoulders.
	(3) 15 Russian Twists	Core, Obliques, Shoulders	Rotate torso holding dumbbell, seated with legs lifted.
21	**5 Rounds for time:**		
	(1) 10 Thrusters	Shoulders, Legs, Core	Squat down, then press dumbbells overhead in one motion.
	(2) 15 Renegade Rows	Back, Shoulders, Core	Row dumbbell from plank position, alternating sides.
	(3) 20 Russian Twists	Core, Obliques, Shoulders	Rotate torso holding dumbbell, seated with legs lifted.

Workout No.		Workout (Dumbbell Exercises only)	Main Muscle Groups	Instructions
22		**As many rounds as possible in 12 mins of:**		
	(1)	10 Goblet Squats	Legs, Glutes, Core	Hold dumbbell at chest, perform deep squat.
	(2)	15 Single Arm Rows (each side)	Back, Biceps, Core	Row dumbbell to hip while bent over, switch sides.
	(3)	20 Hammer Curls	Biceps, Forearms	Curl dumbbells with palms facing each other.
23		**4 Rounds for time:**		
	(1)	12 Step-Ups (each leg)	Legs, Glutes, Core	Step onto platform holding dumbbells, alternating legs.
	(2)	15 Shoulder Presses	Shoulders, Triceps	Press dumbbells overhead from shoulders.
	(3)	20 V-Sit Cross Jabs	Core, Shoulders, Arms	Sit in V position, punch across body with dumbbell.
24		**Every minute on the minute for 20 mins:**		
	(1)	5 Jump Squats	Legs, Glutes, Core	Perform squat then jump, holding dumbbells.
	(2)	10 Bench Presses	Chest, Shoulders, Triceps	Press dumbbells from chest to straight arms on a bench.
	(3)	15 Russian Twists	Core, Obliques, Shoulders	Rotate torso holding dumbbell, seated with legs lifted.
25		**5 Rounds for time:**		
	(1)	10 Sumo Squats	Legs, Glutes, Core	Squat with wide stance, holding dumbbell.
	(2)	12 Seesaw Rows	Back, Biceps, Core	Row one dumbbell while other lowers, alternating.
	(3)	15 Plank Ts	Core, Shoulders, Arms	Rotate into T position from plank with dumbbell.
26		**45 secs work / 15 secs rest per exercise for 4 rounds:**		
	(1)	Dumbbell Swing	Legs, Core, Shoulders	Swing dumbbell between legs then up to shoulder height.
	(2)	Reverse Fly	Shoulders, Upper Back	Lift dumbbells outward while bent over.
	(3)	Calf Raise	Calves, Legs	Lift heels off the ground while holding dumbbells.
27		**20 mins AMRAP (as many rounds as possible):**		
	(1)	10 Alternating Front Raises	Shoulders, Core	Lift dumbbells to shoulder height, alternating arms.
	(2)	12 Glute Bridges	Glutes, Hamstrings, Core	Lift hips while holding dumbbell on hips.
	(3)	15 Concentration Curls	Biceps	Curl dumbbell with elbow on thigh, focus on bicep.
28		**30 secs work / 30 secs rest per exercise for 5 rounds:**		
	(1)	Farmer's Walk	Shoulders, Core, Legs	Walk holding heavy dumbbells at sides.
	(2)	Reverse Lunge	Legs, Glutes, Core	Step back into lunge, holding dumbbells at sides.
	(3)	Side Raise	Shoulders, Core	Lift dumbbells to sides, shoulder height.

Workout No.	Workout (Dumbbell Exercises only)	Main Muscle Groups	Instructions
29	**4 Rounds for time:**		
	(1) 10 Romanian Deadlifts	Hamstrings, Glutes, Lower Back	Lower dumbbells to shins with slight knee bend, then lift.
	(2) 12 Tricep Extensions	Triceps, Shoulders	Extend dumbbell overhead, bending elbow.
	(3) 15 Floor T Raises	Shoulders, Upper Back	Lift dumbbells to form T-shape while lying face down.
30	**Every minute on the minute for 16 mins:**		
	(1) 5 Goblet Squats	Legs, Glutes, Core	Hold dumbbell at chest, perform deep squat.
	(2) 10 Shoulder Presses	Shoulders, Triceps	Press dumbbells overhead from shoulders.
	(3) 15 Russian Twists	Core, Obliques, Shoulders	Rotate torso holding dumbbell, seated with legs lifted.
31	**5 Rounds for time:**		
	(1) 15 Dumbbell Pullover	Chest, Back, Core	Lower dumbbell behind head while lying on bench, then lift.
	(2) 10 Tricep Kickbacks (each arm)	Triceps, Shoulders	Extend arm backward holding dumbbell from bent-over position.
	(3) 20 Jump Squats	Legs, Glutes, Core	Perform squat then jump, holding dumbbells.
32	**As many rounds as possible in 15 mins of:**		
	(1) 12 Goblet Squats	Legs, Glutes, Core	Hold dumbbell at chest, perform deep squat.
	(2) 10 Renegade Rows	Back, Shoulders, Core	Row dumbbell from plank position, alternating sides.
	(3) 15 Russian Twists	Core, Obliques, Shoulders	Rotate torso holding dumbbell, seated with legs lifted.
33	**4 Rounds for time:**		
	(1) 10 Thrusters	Shoulders, Legs, Core	Squat down, then press dumbbells overhead in one motion.
	(2) 12 Single Arm Rows (each side)	Back, Biceps, Core	Row dumbbell to hip while bent over, switch sides.
	(3) 20 Concentration Curls	Biceps	Curl dumbbell with elbow on thigh, focus on bicep.
34	**Every minute on the minute for 18 mins:**		
	(1) 10 Bench Presses	Chest, Shoulders, Triceps	Press dumbbells from chest to straight arms on a bench.
	(2) 12 Side Raises	Shoulders, Core	Lift dumbbells to sides, shoulder height.
	(3) 15 V-Sit Cross Jabs	Core, Shoulders, Arms	Sit in V position, punch across body with dumbbell.
35	**5 Rounds for time:**		
	(1) 10 Sumo Squats	Legs, Glutes, Core	Squat with wide stance, holding dumbbell.
	(2) 15 Shoulder Shrugs	Shoulders, Traps	Lift shoulders toward ears holding dumbbells.
	(3) 20 Hammer Curls	Biceps, Forearms	Curl dumbbells with palms facing each other.

Workout No.	Workout (Dumbbell Exercises only)	Main Muscle Groups	Instructions
36	**45 secs work / 15 secs rest per exercise for 4 rounds:**		
	(1) Dumbbell Swing	Legs, Core, Shoulders	Swing dumbbell between legs then up to shoulder height.
	(2) Reverse Fly	Shoulders, Upper Back	Lift dumbbells outward while bent over.
	(3) Calf Raise	Calves, Legs	Lift heels off the ground while holding dumbbells.
37	**20 mins AMRAP (as many rounds as possible):**		
	(1) 10 Alternating Front Raises	Shoulders, Core	Lift dumbbells to shoulder height, alternating arms.
	(2) 12 Glute Bridges	Glutes, Hamstrings, Core	Lift hips while holding dumbbell on hips.
	(3) 15 Concentration Curls	Biceps	Curl dumbbell with elbow on thigh, focus on bicep.
38	**30 secs work / 30 secs rest per exercise for 5 rounds:**		
	(1) Farmer's Walk	Shoulders, Core, Legs	Walk holding heavy dumbbells at sides.
	(2) Reverse Lunge	Legs, Glutes, Core	Step back into lunge, holding dumbbells at sides.
	(3) Side Raise	Shoulders, Core	Lift dumbbells to sides, shoulder height.
39	**4 Rounds for time:**		
	(1) 10 Romanian Deadlifts	Hamstrings, Glutes, Lower Back	Lower dumbbells to shins with slight knee bend, then lift.
	(2) 12 Tricep Extensions	Triceps, Shoulders	Extend dumbbell overhead, bending elbow.
	(3) 15 Floor T Raises	Shoulders, Upper Back	Lift dumbbells to form T-shape while lying face down.
40	**Every minute on the minute for 16 mins:**		
	(1) 5 Goblet Squats	Legs, Glutes, Core	Hold dumbbell at chest, perform deep squat.
	(2) 10 Shoulder Presses	Shoulders, Triceps	Press dumbbells overhead from shoulders.
	(3) 15 Russian Twists	Core, Obliques, Shoulders	Rotate torso holding dumbbell, seated with legs lifted.
41	**5 Rounds for time:**		
	(1) 10 Thrusters	Shoulders, Legs, Core	Squat down, then press dumbbells overhead in one motion.
	(2) 15 Renegade Rows	Back, Shoulders, Core	Row dumbbell from plank position, alternating sides.
	(3) 20 Russian Twists	Core, Obliques, Shoulders	Rotate torso holding dumbbell, seated with legs lifted.
42	**As many rounds as possible in 12 mins of:**		
	(1) 10 Goblet Squats	Legs, Glutes, Core	Hold dumbbell at chest, perform deep squat.
	(2) 15 Single Arm Rows (each side)	Back, Biceps, Core	Row dumbbell to hip while bent over, switch sides.
	(3) 20 Hammer Curls	Biceps, Forearms	Curl dumbbells with palms facing each other.

Workout No.	Workout (Dumbbell Exercises only)	Main Muscle Groups	Instructions
43	**4 Rounds for time:**		
	(1) 12 Step-Ups (each leg)	Legs, Glutes, Core	Step onto platform holding dumbbells, alternating legs.
	(2) 15 Shoulder Presses	Shoulders, Triceps	Press dumbbells overhead from shoulders.
	(3) 20 V-Sit Cross Jabs	Core, Shoulders, Arms	Sit in V position, punch across body with dumbbell.
44	**Every minute on the minute for 20 mins:**		
	(1) 5 Jump Squats	Legs, Glutes, Core	Perform squat then jump, holding dumbbells.
	(2) 10 Bench Presses	Chest, Shoulders, Triceps	Press dumbbells from chest to straight arms on a bench.
	(3) 15 Russian Twists	Core, Obliques, Shoulders	Rotate torso holding dumbbell, seated with legs lifted.
45	**5 Rounds for time:**		
	(1) 10 Sumo Squats	Legs, Glutes, Core	Squat with wide stance, holding dumbbell.
	(2) 12 Seesaw Rows	Back, Biceps, Core	Row one dumbbell while other lowers, alternating.
	(3) 15 Plank Ts	Core, Shoulders, Arms	Rotate into T position from plank with dumbbell.
46	**45 secs work / 15 secs rest per exercise for 4 rounds:**		
	(1) Dumbbell Swing	Legs, Core, Shoulders	Swing dumbbell between legs then up to shoulder height.
	(2) Reverse Fly	Shoulders, Upper Back	Lift dumbbells outward while bent over.
	(3) Calf Raise	Calves, Legs	Lift heels off the ground while holding dumbbells.
47	**20 mins AMRAP (as many rounds as possible):**		
	(1) 10 Alternating Front Raises	Shoulders, Core	Lift dumbbells to shoulder height, alternating arms.
	(2) 12 Glute Bridges	Glutes, Hamstrings, Core	Lift hips while holding dumbbell on hips.
	(3) 15 Concentration Curls	Biceps	Curl dumbbell with elbow on thigh, focus on bicep.
48	**30 secs work / 30 secs rest per exercise for 5 rounds:**		
	(1) Farmer's Walk	Shoulders, Core, Legs	Walk holding heavy dumbbells at sides.
	(2) Reverse Lunge	Legs, Glutes, Core	Step back into lunge, holding dumbbells at sides.
	(3) Side Raise	Shoulders, Core	Lift dumbbells to sides, shoulder height.
49	**4 Rounds for time:**		
	(1) 10 Romanian Deadlifts	Hamstrings, Glutes, Lower Back	Lower dumbbells to shins with slight knee bend, then lift.
	(2) 12 Tricep Extensions	Triceps, Shoulders	Extend dumbbell overhead, bending elbow.
	(3) 15 Floor T Raises	Shoulders, Upper Back	Lift dumbbells to form T-shape while lying face down.

Workout No.	Workout (Dumbbell Exercises only)	Main Muscle Groups	Instructions
50	Every minute on the minute for 16 mins:		
	(1) 5 Goblet Squats	Legs, Glutes, Core	Hold dumbbell at chest, perform deep squat.
	(2) 10 Shoulder Presses	Shoulders, Triceps	Press dumbbells overhead from shoulders.
	(3) 15 Russian Twists	Core, Obliques, Shoulders	Rotate torso holding dumbbell, seated with legs lifted.
51	5 Rounds for time:		
	(1) 10 Thrusters	Shoulders, Legs, Core	Squat down, then press dumbbells overhead in one motion.
	(2) 15 Renegade Rows	Back, Shoulders, Core	Row dumbbell from plank position, alternating sides.
	(3) 20 Russian Twists	Core, Obliques, Shoulders	Rotate torso holding dumbbell, seated with legs lifted.
52	As many rounds as possible in 12 mins of:		
	(1) 10 Goblet Squats	Legs, Glutes, Core	Hold dumbbell at chest, perform deep squat.
	(2) 15 Single Arm Rows (each side)	Back, Biceps, Core	Row dumbbell to hip while bent over, switch sides.
	(3) 20 Hammer Curls	Biceps, Forearms	Curl dumbbells with palms facing each other.
53	4 Rounds for time:		
	(1) 12 Step-Ups (each leg)	Legs, Glutes, Core	Step onto platform holding dumbbells, alternating legs.
	(2) 15 Shoulder Presses	Shoulders, Triceps	Press dumbbells overhead from shoulders.
	(3) 20 V-Sit Cross Jabs	Core, Shoulders, Arms	Sit in V position, punch across body with dumbbell.
54	Every minute on the minute for 20 mins:		
	(1) 5 Jump Squats	Legs, Glutes, Core	Perform squat then jump, holding dumbbells.
	(2) 10 Bench Presses	Chest, Shoulders, Triceps	Press dumbbells from chest to straight arms on a bench.
	(3) 15 Russian Twists	Core, Obliques, Shoulders	Rotate torso holding dumbbell, seated with legs lifted.
55	5 Rounds for time:		
	(1) 10 Sumo Squats	Legs, Glutes, Core	Squat with wide stance, holding dumbbell.
	(2) 12 Seesaw Rows	Back, Biceps, Core	Row one dumbbell while other lowers, alternating.
	(3) 15 Plank Ts	Core, Shoulders, Arms	Rotate into T position from plank with dumbbell.
56	45 secs work / 15 secs rest per exercise for 4 rounds:		
	(1) Dumbbell Swing	Legs, Core, Shoulders	Swing dumbbell between legs then up to shoulder height.
	(2) Reverse Fly	Shoulders, Upper Back	Lift dumbbells outward while bent over.
	(3) Calf Raise	Calves, Legs	Lift heels off the ground while holding dumbbells.

Workout No.		Workout (Dumbbell Exercises only)	Main Muscle Groups	Instructions
57		20 mins AMRAP (as many rounds as possible):		
	(1)	10 Alternating Front Raises	Shoulders, Core	Lift dumbbells to shoulder height, alternating arms.
	(2)	12 Glute Bridges	Glutes, Hamstrings, Core	Lift hips while holding dumbbell on hips.
	(3)	15 Concentration Curls	Biceps	Curl dumbbell with elbow on thigh, focus on bicep.
58		30 secs work / 30 secs rest per exercise for 5 rounds:		
	(1)	Farmer's Walk	Shoulders, Core, Legs	Walk holding heavy dumbbells at sides.
	(2)	Reverse Lunge	Legs, Glutes, Core	Step back into lunge, holding dumbbells at sides.
	(3)	Side Raise	Shoulders, Core	Lift dumbbells to sides, shoulder height.
59		4 Rounds for time:		
	(1)	10 Romanian Deadlifts	Hamstrings, Glutes, Lower Back	Lower dumbbells to shins with slight knee bend, then lift.
	(2)	12 Tricep Extensions	Triceps, Shoulders	Extend dumbbell overhead, bending elbow.
	(3)	15 Floor T Raises	Shoulders, Upper Back	Lift dumbbells to form T-shape while lying face down.
60		Every minute on the minute for 16 mins:		
	(1)	5 Goblet Squats	Legs, Glutes, Core	Hold dumbbell at chest, perform deep squat.
	(2)	10 Shoulder Presses	Shoulders, Triceps	Press dumbbells overhead from shoulders.
	(3)	15 Russian Twists	Core, Obliques, Shoulders	Rotate torso holding dumbbell, seated with legs lifted.
61		5 Rounds for time:		
	(1)	10 Thrusters	Shoulders, Legs, Core	Squat down, then press dumbbells overhead in one motion.
	(2)	15 Renegade Rows	Back, Shoulders, Core	Row dumbbell from plank position, alternating sides.
	(3)	20 Russian Twists	Core, Obliques, Shoulders	Rotate torso holding dumbbell, seated with legs lifted.
62		As many rounds as possible in 12 mins of:		
	(1)	10 Goblet Squats	Legs, Glutes, Core	Hold dumbbell at chest, perform deep squat.
	(2)	15 Single Arm Rows (each side)	Back, Biceps, Core	Row dumbbell to hip while bent over, switch sides.
	(3)	20 Hammer Curls	Biceps, Forearms	Curl dumbbells with palms facing each other.
63		4 Rounds for time:		
	(1)	12 Step-Ups (each leg)	Legs, Glutes, Core	Step onto platform holding dumbbells, alternating legs.
	(2)	15 Shoulder Presses	Shoulders, Triceps	Press dumbbells overhead from shoulders.
	(3)	20 V-Sit Cross Jabs	Core, Shoulders, Arms	Sit in V position, punch across body with dumbbell.

Workout No.	Workout (Dumbbell Exercises only)	Main Muscle Groups	Instructions
64	**Every minute on the minute for 20 mins:**		
	(1) 5 Jump Squats	Legs, Glutes, Core	Perform squat then jump, holding dumbbells.
	(2) 10 Bench Presses	Chest, Shoulders, Triceps	Press dumbbells from chest to straight arms on a bench.
	(3) 15 Russian Twists	Core, Obliques, Shoulders	Rotate torso holding dumbbell, seated with legs lifted.
65	**5 Rounds for time:**		
	(1) 10 Sumo Squats	Legs, Glutes, Core	Squat with wide stance, holding dumbbell.
	(2) 12 Seesaw Rows	Back, Biceps, Core	Row one dumbbell while other lowers, alternating.
	(3) 15 Plank Ts	Core, Shoulders, Arms	Rotate into T position from plank with dumbbell.
66	**45 secs work / 15 secs rest per exercise for 4 rounds:**		
	(1) Dumbbell Swing	Legs, Core, Shoulders	Swing dumbbell between legs then up to shoulder height.
	(2) Reverse Fly	Shoulders, Upper Back	Lift dumbbells outward while bent over.
	(3) Calf Raise	Calves, Legs	Lift heels off the ground while holding dumbbells.
67	**20 mins AMRAP (as many rounds as possible):**		
	(1) 10 Alternating Front Raises	Shoulders, Core	Lift dumbbells to shoulder height, alternating arms.
	(2) 12 Glute Bridges	Glutes, Hamstrings, Core	Lift hips while holding dumbbell on hips.
	(3) 15 Concentration Curls	Biceps	Curl dumbbell with elbow on thigh, focus on bicep.
68	**30 secs work / 30 secs rest per exercise for 5 rounds:**		
	(1) Farmer's Walk	Shoulders, Core, Legs	Walk holding heavy dumbbells at sides.
	(2) Reverse Lunge	Legs, Glutes, Core	Step back into lunge, holding dumbbells at sides.
	(3) Side Raise	Shoulders, Core	Lift dumbbells to sides, shoulder height.
69	**4 Rounds for time:**		
	(1) 10 Romanian Deadlifts	Hamstrings, Glutes, Lower Back	Lower dumbbells to shins with slight knee bend, then lift.
	(2) 12 Tricep Extensions	Triceps, Shoulders	Extend dumbbell overhead, bending elbow.
	(3) 15 Floor T Raises	Shoulders, Upper Back	Lift dumbbells to form T-shape while lying face down.
70	**Every minute on the minute for 16 mins:**		
	(1) 5 Goblet Squats	Legs, Glutes, Core	Hold dumbbell at chest, perform deep squat.
	(2) 10 Shoulder Presses	Shoulders, Triceps	Press dumbbells overhead from shoulders.
	(3) 15 Russian Twists	Core, Obliques, Shoulders	Rotate torso holding dumbbell, seated with legs lifted.

Workout No.		Workout (Dumbbell Exercises only)	Main Muscle Groups	Instructions
71		**5 Rounds for time:**		
	(1)	10 Thrusters	Shoulders, Legs, Core	Squat down, then press dumbbells overhead in one motion.
	(2)	15 Renegade Rows	Back, Shoulders, Core	Row dumbbell from plank position, alternating sides.
	(3)	20 Russian Twists	Core, Obliques, Shoulders	Rotate torso holding dumbbell, seated with legs lifted.
72		**As many rounds as possible in 12 mins of:**		
	(1)	10 Goblet Squats	Legs, Glutes, Core	Hold dumbbell at chest, perform deep squat.
	(2)	15 Single Arm Rows (each side)	Back, Biceps, Core	Row dumbbell to hip while bent over, switch sides.
	(3)	20 Hammer Curls	Biceps, Forearms	Curl dumbbells with palms facing each other.
73		**4 Rounds for time:**		
	(1)	12 Step-Ups (each leg)	Legs, Glutes, Core	Step onto platform holding dumbbells, alternating legs.
	(2)	15 Shoulder Presses	Shoulders, Triceps	Press dumbbells overhead from shoulders.
	(3)	20 V-Sit Cross Jabs	Core, Shoulders, Arms	Sit in V position, punch across body with dumbbell.
74		**Every minute on the minute for 20 mins:**		
	(1)	5 Jump Squats	Legs, Glutes, Core	Perform squat then jump, holding dumbbells.
	(2)	10 Bench Presses	Chest, Shoulders, Triceps	Press dumbbells from chest to straight arms on a bench.
	(3)	15 Russian Twists	Core, Obliques, Shoulders	Rotate torso holding dumbbell, seated with legs lifted.
75		**5 Rounds for time:**		
	(1)	10 Sumo Squats	Legs, Glutes, Core	Squat with wide stance, holding dumbbell.
	(2)	12 Seesaw Rows	Back, Biceps, Core	Row one dumbbell while other lowers, alternating.
	(3)	15 Plank Ts	Core, Shoulders, Arms	Rotate into T position from plank with dumbbell.
76		**45 secs work / 15 secs rest per exercise for 4 rounds:**		
	(1)	Dumbbell Swing	Legs, Core, Shoulders	Swing dumbbell between legs then up to shoulder height.
	(2)	Reverse Fly	Shoulders, Upper Back	Lift dumbbells outward while bent over.
	(3)	Calf Raise	Calves, Legs	Lift heels off the ground while holding dumbbells.
77		**20 mins AMRAP (as many rounds as possible):**		
	(1)	10 Alternating Front Raises	Shoulders, Core	Lift dumbbells to shoulder height, alternating arms.
	(2)	12 Glute Bridges	Glutes, Hamstrings, Core	Lift hips while holding dumbbell on hips.
	(3)	15 Concentration Curls	Biceps	Curl dumbbell with elbow on thigh, focus on bicep.

Workout No.	Workout (Dumbbell Exercises only)	Main Muscle Groups	Instructions
78	**30 secs work / 30 secs rest per exercise for 5 rounds:**		
	(1) Farmer's Walk	Shoulders, Core, Legs	Walk holding heavy dumbbells at sides.
	(2) Reverse Lunge	Legs, Glutes, Core	Step back into lunge, holding dumbbells at sides.
	(3) Side Raise	Shoulders, Core	Lift dumbbells to sides, shoulder height.
79	**4 Rounds for time:**		
	(1) 10 Romanian Deadlifts	Hamstrings, Glutes, Lower Back	Lower dumbbells to shins with slight knee bend, then lift.
	(2) 12 Tricep Extensions	Triceps, Shoulders	Extend dumbbell overhead, bending elbow.
	(3) 15 Floor T Raises	Shoulders, Upper Back	Lift dumbbells to form T-shape while lying face down.
80	**Every minute on the minute for 16 mins:**		
	(1) 5 Goblet Squats	Legs, Glutes, Core	Hold dumbbell at chest, perform deep squat.
	(2) 10 Shoulder Presses	Shoulders, Triceps	Press dumbbells overhead from shoulders.
	(3) 15 Russian Twists	Core, Obliques, Shoulders	Rotate torso holding dumbbell, seated with legs lifted.
81	**5 Rounds for time:**		
	(1) 10 Thrusters	Shoulders, Legs, Core	Squat down, then press dumbbells overhead in one motion.
	(2) 15 Renegade Rows	Back, Shoulders, Core	Row dumbbell from plank position, alternating sides.
	(3) 20 Russian Twists	Core, Obliques, Shoulders	Rotate torso holding dumbbell, seated with legs lifted.
82	**As many rounds as possible in 12 mins of:**		
	(1) 10 Goblet Squats	Legs, Glutes, Core	Hold dumbbell at chest, perform deep squat.
	(2) 15 Single Arm Rows (each side)	Back, Biceps, Core	Row dumbbell to hip while bent over, switch sides.
	(3) 20 Hammer Curls	Biceps, Forearms	Curl dumbbells with palms facing each other.
83	**4 Rounds for time:**		
	(1) 12 Step-Ups (each leg)	Legs, Glutes, Core	Step onto platform holding dumbbells, alternating legs.
	(2) 15 Shoulder Presses	Shoulders, Triceps	Press dumbbells overhead from shoulders.
	(3) 20 V-Sit Cross Jabs	Core, Shoulders, Arms	Sit in V position, punch across body with dumbbell.
84	**Every minute on the minute for 20 mins:**		
	(1) 5 Jump Squats	Legs, Glutes, Core	Perform squat then jump, holding dumbbells.
	(2) 10 Bench Presses	Chest, Shoulders, Triceps	Press dumbbells from chest to straight arms on a bench.
	(3) 15 Russian Twists	Core, Obliques, Shoulders	Rotate torso holding dumbbell, seated with legs lifted.

Workout No.	Workout (Dumbbell Exercises only)	Main Muscle Groups	Instructions
85	**5 Rounds for time:**		
	(1) 10 Sumo Squats	Legs, Glutes, Core	Squat with wide stance, holding dumbbell.
	(2) 12 Seesaw Rows	Back, Biceps, Core	Row one dumbbell while other lowers, alternating.
	(3) 15 Plank Ts	Core, Shoulders, Arms	Rotate into T position from plank with dumbbell.
86	**45 secs work / 15 secs rest per exercise for 4 rounds:**		
	(1) Dumbbell Swing	Legs, Core, Shoulders	Swing dumbbell between legs then up to shoulder height.
	(2) Reverse Fly	Shoulders, Upper Back	Lift dumbbells outward while bent over.
	(3) Calf Raise	Calves, Legs	Lift heels off the ground while holding dumbbells.
87	**20 mins AMRAP (as many rounds as possible):**		
	(1) 10 Alternating Front Raises	Shoulders, Core	Lift dumbbells to shoulder height, alternating arms.
	(2) 12 Glute Bridges	Glutes, Hamstrings, Core	Lift hips while holding dumbbell on hips.
	(3) 15 Concentration Curls	Biceps	Curl dumbbell with elbow on thigh, focus on bicep.
88	**30 secs work / 30 secs rest per exercise for 5 rounds:**		
	(1) Farmer's Walk	Shoulders, Core, Legs	Walk holding heavy dumbbells at sides.
	(2) Reverse Lunge	Legs, Glutes, Core	Step back into lunge, holding dumbbells at sides.
	(3) Side Raise	Shoulders, Core	Lift dumbbells to sides, shoulder height.
89	**4 Rounds for time:**		
	(1) 10 Romanian Deadlifts	Hamstrings, Glutes, Lower Back	Lower dumbbells to shins with slight knee bend, then lift.
	(2) 12 Tricep Extensions	Triceps, Shoulders	Extend dumbbell overhead, bending elbow.
	(3) 15 Floor T Raises	Shoulders, Upper Back	Lift dumbbells to form T-shape while lying face down.
90	**Every minute on the minute for 16 mins:**		
	(1) 5 Goblet Squats	Legs, Glutes, Core	Hold dumbbell at chest, perform deep squat.
	(2) 10 Shoulder Presses	Shoulders, Triceps	Press dumbbells overhead from shoulders.
	(3) 15 Russian Twists	Core, Obliques, Shoulders	Rotate torso holding dumbbell, seated with legs lifted.
91	**5 Rounds for time:**		
	(1) 10 Thrusters	Shoulders, Legs, Core	Squat down, then press dumbbells overhead in one motion.
	(2) 15 Renegade Rows	Back, Shoulders, Core	Row dumbbell from plank position, alternating sides.
	(3) 20 Russian Twists	Core, Obliques, Shoulders	Rotate torso holding dumbbell, seated with legs lifted.

Workout No.	Workout (Dumbbell Exercises only)	Main Muscle Groups	Instructions
92	As many rounds as possible in 12 mins of:		
(1)	10 Goblet Squats	Legs, Glutes, Core	Hold dumbbell at chest, perform deep squat.
(2)	15 Single Arm Rows (each side)	Back, Biceps, Core	Row dumbbell to hip while bent over, switch sides.
(3)	20 Hammer Curls	Biceps, Forearms	Curl dumbbells with palms facing each other.
93	4 Rounds for time:		
(1)	12 Step-Ups (each leg)	Legs, Glutes, Core	Step onto platform holding dumbbells, alternating legs.
(2)	15 Shoulder Presses	Shoulders, Triceps	Press dumbbells overhead from shoulders.
(3)	20 V-Sit Cross Jabs	Core, Shoulders, Arms	Sit in V position, punch across body with dumbbell.
94	Every minute on the minute for 20 mins:		
(1)	5 Jump Squats	Legs, Glutes, Core	Perform squat then jump, holding dumbbells.
(2)	10 Bench Presses	Chest, Shoulders, Triceps	Press dumbbells from chest to straight arms on a bench.
(3)	15 Russian Twists	Core, Obliques, Shoulders	Rotate torso holding dumbbell, seated with legs lifted.
95	5 Rounds for time:		
(1)	10 Sumo Squats	Legs, Glutes, Core	Squat with wide stance, holding dumbbell.
(2)	12 Seesaw Rows	Back, Biceps, Core	Row one dumbbell while other lowers, alternating.
(3)	15 Plank Ts	Core, Shoulders, Arms	Rotate into T position from plank with dumbbell.
96	45 secs work / 15 secs rest per exercise for 4 rounds:		
(1)	Dumbbell Swing	Legs, Core, Shoulders	Swing dumbbell between legs then up to shoulder height.
(2)	Reverse Fly	Shoulders, Upper Back	Lift dumbbells outward while bent over.
(3)	Calf Raise	Calves, Legs	Lift heels off the ground while holding dumbbells.
97	20 mins AMRAP (as many rounds as possible):		
(1)	10 Alternating Front Raises	Shoulders, Core	Lift dumbbells to shoulder height, alternating arms.
(2)	12 Glute Bridges	Glutes, Hamstrings, Core	Lift hips while holding dumbbell on hips.
(3)	15 Concentration Curls	Biceps	Curl dumbbell with elbow on thigh, focus on bicep.
98	30 secs work / 30 secs rest per exercise for 5 rounds:		
(1)	Farmer's Walk	Shoulders, Core, Legs	Walk holding heavy dumbbells at sides.
(2)	Reverse Lunge	Legs, Glutes, Core	Step back into lunge, holding dumbbells at sides.
(3)	Side Raise	Shoulders, Core	Lift dumbbells to sides, shoulder height.

Workout No.	Workout (Dumbbell Exercises only)		Main Muscle Groups	Instructions
99	4 Rounds for time:			
	(1)	10 Romanian Deadlifts	Hamstrings, Glutes, Lower Back	Lower dumbbells to shins with slight knee bend, then lift.
	(2)	12 Tricep Extensions	Triceps, Shoulders	Extend dumbbell overhead, bending elbow.
	(3)	15 Floor T Raises	Shoulders, Upper Back	Lift dumbbells to form T-shape while lying face down.
100	Every minute on the minute for 16 mins:			
	(1)	5 Goblet Squats	Legs, Glutes, Core	Hold dumbbell at chest, perform deep squat.
	(2)	10 Shoulder Presses	Shoulders, Triceps	Press dumbbells overhead from shoulders.
	(3)	15 Russian Twists	Core, Obliques, Shoulders	Rotate torso holding dumbbell, seated with legs lifted.
101	5 Rounds for time:			
	(1)	10 Thrusters	Shoulders, Legs, Core	Squat down, then press dumbbells overhead in one motion.
	(2)	15 Single Arm Rows (each side)	Back, Biceps, Core	Row dumbbell to hip while bent over, switch sides.
	(3)	20 Russian Twists	Core, Obliques, Shoulders	Rotate torso holding dumbbell, seated with legs lifted.
102	As many rounds as possible in 12 mins of:			
	(1)	10 Goblet Squats	Legs, Glutes, Core	Hold dumbbell at chest, perform deep squat.
	(2)	15 Renegade Rows	Back, Shoulders, Core	Row dumbbell from plank position, alternating sides.
	(3)	20 Hammer Curls	Biceps, Forearms	Curl dumbbells with palms facing each other.
103	4 Rounds for time:			
	(1)	12 Step-Ups (each leg)	Legs, Glutes, Core	Step onto platform holding dumbbells, alternating legs.
	(2)	15 Shoulder Presses	Shoulders, Triceps	Press dumbbells overhead from shoulders.
	(3)	20 V-Sit Cross Jabs	Core, Shoulders, Arms	Sit in V position, punch across body with dumbbell.
104	Every minute on the minute for 20 mins:			
	(1)	5 Jump Squats	Legs, Glutes, Core	Perform squat then jump, holding dumbbells.
	(2)	10 Bench Presses	Chest, Shoulders, Triceps	Press dumbbells from chest to straight arms on a bench.
	(3)	15 Russian Twists	Core, Obliques, Shoulders	Rotate torso holding dumbbell, seated with legs lifted.
105	5 Rounds for time:			
	(1)	10 Sumo Squats	Legs, Glutes, Core	Squat with wide stance, holding dumbbell.
	(2)	12 Seesaw Rows	Back, Biceps, Core	Row one dumbbell while other lowers, alternating.
	(3)	15 Plank Ts	Core, Shoulders, Arms	Rotate into T position from plank with dumbbell.

Workout No.	Workout (Dumbbell Exercises only)	Main Muscle Groups	Instructions
106	**45 secs work / 15 secs rest per exercise for 4 rounds:**		
	(1) Dumbbell Swing	Legs, Core, Shoulders	Swing dumbbell between legs then up to shoulder height.
	(2) Reverse Fly	Shoulders, Upper Back	Lift dumbbells outward while bent over.
	(3) Calf Raise	Calves, Legs	Lift heels off the ground while holding dumbbells.
107	**20 mins AMRAP (as many rounds as possible):**		
	(1) 10 Alternating Front Raises	Shoulders, Core	Lift dumbbells to shoulder height, alternating arms.
	(2) 12 Glute Bridges	Glutes, Hamstrings, Core	Lift hips while holding dumbbell on hips.
	(3) 15 Concentration Curls	Biceps	Curl dumbbell with elbow on thigh, focus on bicep.
108	**30 secs work / 30 secs rest per exercise for 5 rounds:**		
	(1) Farmer's Walk	Shoulders, Core, Legs	Walk holding heavy dumbbells at sides.
	(2) Reverse Lunge	Legs, Glutes, Core	Step back into lunge, holding dumbbells at sides.
	(3) Side Raise	Shoulders, Core	Lift dumbbells to sides, shoulder height.
109	**4 Rounds for time:**		
	(1) 10 Romanian Deadlifts	Hamstrings, Glutes, Lower Back	Lower dumbbells to shins with slight knee bend, then lift.
	(2) 12 Tricep Extensions	Triceps, Shoulders	Extend dumbbell overhead, bending elbow.
	(3) 15 Floor T Raises	Shoulders, Upper Back	Lift dumbbells to form T-shape while lying face down.
110	**Every minute on the minute for 16 mins:**		
	(1) 5 Goblet Squats	Legs, Glutes, Core	Hold dumbbell at chest, perform deep squat.
	(2) 10 Shoulder Presses	Shoulders, Triceps	Press dumbbells overhead from shoulders.
	(3) 15 Russian Twists	Core, Obliques, Shoulders	Rotate torso holding dumbbell, seated with legs lifted.
111	**5 Rounds for time:**		
	(1) 10 Thrusters	Shoulders, Legs, Core	Squat down, then press dumbbells overhead in one motion.
	(2) 15 Renegade Rows	Back, Shoulders, Core	Row dumbbell from plank position, alternating sides.
	(3) 20 Russian Twists	Core, Obliques, Shoulders	Rotate torso holding dumbbell, seated with legs lifted.
112	**As many rounds as possible in 12 mins of:**		
	(1) 10 Goblet Squats	Legs, Glutes, Core	Hold dumbbell at chest, perform deep squat.
	(2) 15 Single Arm Rows (each side)	Back, Biceps, Core	Row dumbbell to hip while bent over, switch sides.
	(3) 20 Hammer Curls	Biceps, Forearms	Curl dumbbells with palms facing each other.

Workout No.	Workout (Dumbbell Exercises only)		Main Muscle Groups	Instructions
113	**4 Rounds for time:**			
	(1)	12 Step-Ups (each leg)	Legs, Glutes, Core	Step onto platform holding dumbbells, alternating legs.
	(2)	15 Shoulder Presses	Shoulders, Triceps	Press dumbbells overhead from shoulders.
	(3)	20 V-Sit Cross Jabs	Core, Shoulders, Arms	Sit in V position, punch across body with dumbbell.
114	**Every minute on the minute for 20 mins:**			
	(1)	5 Jump Squats	Legs, Glutes, Core	Perform squat then jump, holding dumbbells.
	(2)	10 Bench Presses	Chest, Shoulders, Triceps	Press dumbbells from chest to straight arms on a bench.
	(3)	15 Russian Twists	Core, Obliques, Shoulders	Rotate torso holding dumbbell, seated with legs lifted.
115	**5 Rounds for time:**			
	(1)	10 Sumo Squats	Legs, Glutes, Core	Squat with wide stance, holding dumbbell.
	(2)	12 Seesaw Rows	Back, Biceps, Core	Row one dumbbell while other lowers, alternating.
	(3)	15 Plank Ts	Core, Shoulders, Arms	Rotate into T position from plank with dumbbell.
116	**45 secs work / 15 secs rest per exercise for 4 rounds:**			
	(1)	Dumbbell Swing	Legs, Core, Shoulders	Swing dumbbell between legs then up to shoulder height.
	(2)	Reverse Fly	Shoulders, Upper Back	Lift dumbbells outward while bent over.
	(3)	Calf Raise	Calves, Legs	Lift heels off the ground while holding dumbbells.
117	**20 mins AMRAP (as many rounds as possible):**			
	(1)	10 Alternating Front Raises	Shoulders, Core	Lift dumbbells to shoulder height, alternating arms.
	(2)	12 Glute Bridges	Glutes, Hamstrings, Core	Lift hips while holding dumbbell on hips.
	(3)	15 Concentration Curls	Biceps	Curl dumbbell with elbow on thigh, focus on bicep.
118	**30 secs work / 30 secs rest per exercise for 5 rounds:**			
	(1)	Farmer's Walk	Shoulders, Core, Legs	Walk holding heavy dumbbells at sides.
	(2)	Reverse Lunge	Legs, Glutes, Core	Step back into lunge, holding dumbbells at sides.
	(3)	Side Raise	Shoulders, Core	Lift dumbbells to sides, shoulder height.
119	**4 Rounds for time:**			
	(1)	10 Romanian Deadlifts	Hamstrings, Glutes, Lower Back	Lower dumbbells to shins with slight knee bend, then lift.
	(2)	12 Tricep Extensions	Triceps, Shoulders	Extend dumbbell overhead, bending elbow.
	(3)	15 Floor T Raises	Shoulders, Upper Back	Lift dumbbells to form T-shape while lying face down.

Workout No.	Workout (Dumbbell Exercises only)		Main Muscle Groups	Instructions
120	Every minute on the minute for 16 mins:			
	(1)	5 Goblet Squats	Legs, Glutes, Core	Hold dumbbell at chest, perform deep squat.
	(2)	10 Shoulder Presses	Shoulders, Triceps	Press dumbbells overhead from shoulders.
	(3)	15 Russian Twists	Core, Obliques, Shoulders	Rotate torso holding dumbbell, seated with legs lifted.
121	5 Rounds for time:			
	(1)	10 Thrusters	Shoulders, Legs, Core	Squat down, then press dumbbells overhead in one motion.
	(2)	15 Renegade Rows	Back, Shoulders, Core	Row dumbbell from plank position, alternating sides.
	(3)	20 Russian Twists	Core, Obliques, Shoulders	Rotate torso holding dumbbell, seated with legs lifted.
122	As many rounds as possible in 12 mins of:			
	(1)	10 Goblet Squats	Legs, Glutes, Core	Hold dumbbell at chest, perform deep squat.
	(2)	15 Single Arm Rows (each side)	Back, Biceps, Core	Row dumbbell to hip while bent over, switch sides.
	(3)	20 Hammer Curls	Biceps, Forearms	Curl dumbbells with palms facing each other.
123	4 Rounds for time:			
	(1)	12 Step-Ups (each leg)	Legs, Glutes, Core	Step onto platform holding dumbbells, alternating legs.
	(2)	15 Shoulder Presses	Shoulders, Triceps	Press dumbbells overhead from shoulders.
	(3)	20 V-Sit Cross Jabs	Core, Shoulders, Arms	Sit in V position, punch across body with dumbbell.
124	Every minute on the minute for 20 mins:			
	(1)	5 Jump Squats	Legs, Glutes, Core	Perform squat then jump, holding dumbbells.
	(2)	10 Bench Presses	Chest, Shoulders, Triceps	Press dumbbells from chest to straight arms on a bench.
	(3)	15 Russian Twists	Core, Obliques, Shoulders	Rotate torso holding dumbbell, seated with legs lifted.
125	5 Rounds for time:			
	(1)	10 Sumo Squats	Legs, Glutes, Core	Squat with wide stance, holding dumbbell.
	(2)	12 Seesaw Rows	Back, Biceps, Core	Row one dumbbell while other lowers, alternating.
	(3)	15 Plank Ts	Core, Shoulders, Arms	Rotate into T position from plank with dumbbell.
126	45 secs work / 15 secs rest per exercise for 4 rounds:			
	(1)	Dumbbell Swing	Legs, Core, Shoulders	Swing dumbbell between legs then up to shoulder height.
	(2)	Reverse Fly	Shoulders, Upper Back	Lift dumbbells outward while bent over.
	(3)	Calf Raise	Calves, Legs	Lift heels off the ground while holding dumbbells.

Workout No.		Workout (Dumbbell Exercises only)	Main Muscle Groups	Instructions
127		**20 mins AMRAP (as many rounds as possible):**		
	(1)	10 Alternating Front Raises	Shoulders, Core	Lift dumbbells to shoulder height, alternating arms.
	(2)	12 Glute Bridges	Glutes, Hamstrings, Core	Lift hips while holding dumbbell on hips.
	(3)	15 Concentration Curls	Biceps	Curl dumbbell with elbow on thigh, focus on bicep.
128		**30 secs work / 30 secs rest per exercise for 5 rounds:**		
	(1)	Farmer's Walk	Shoulders, Core, Legs	Walk holding heavy dumbbells at sides.
	(2)	Reverse Lunge	Legs, Glutes, Core	Step back into lunge, holding dumbbells at sides.
	(3)	Side Raise	Shoulders, Core	Lift dumbbells to sides, shoulder height.
129		**4 Rounds for time:**		
	(1)	10 Romanian Deadlifts	Hamstrings, Glutes, Lower Back	Lower dumbbells to shins with slight knee bend, then lift.
	(2)	12 Tricep Extensions	Triceps, Shoulders	Extend dumbbell overhead, bending elbow.
	(3)	15 Floor T Raises	Shoulders, Upper Back	Lift dumbbells to form T-shape while lying face down.
130		**Every minute on the minute for 16 mins:**		
	(1)	5 Goblet Squats	Legs, Glutes, Core	Hold dumbbell at chest, perform deep squat.
	(2)	10 Shoulder Presses	Shoulders, Triceps	Press dumbbells overhead from shoulders.
	(3)	15 Russian Twists	Core, Obliques, Shoulders	Rotate torso holding dumbbell, seated with legs lifted.
131		**5 Rounds for time:**		
	(1)	10 Thrusters	Shoulders, Legs, Core	Squat down, then press dumbbells overhead in one motion.
	(2)	15 Renegade Rows	Back, Shoulders, Core	Row dumbbell from plank position, alternating sides.
	(3)	20 Russian Twists	Core, Obliques, Shoulders	Rotate torso holding dumbbell, seated with legs lifted.
132		**As many rounds as possible in 12 mins of:**		
	(1)	10 Goblet Squats	Legs, Glutes, Core	Hold dumbbell at chest, perform deep squat.
	(2)	15 Single Arm Rows (each side)	Back, Biceps, Core	Row dumbbell to hip while bent over, switch sides.
	(3)	20 Hammer Curls	Biceps, Forearms	Curl dumbbells with palms facing each other.
133		**4 Rounds for time:**		
	(1)	12 Step-Ups (each leg)	Legs, Glutes, Core	Step onto platform holding dumbbells, alternating legs.
	(2)	15 Shoulder Presses	Shoulders, Triceps	Press dumbbells overhead from shoulders.
	(3)	20 V-Sit Cross Jabs	Core, Shoulders, Arms	Sit in V position, punch across body with dumbbell.

Workout No.	Workout (Dumbbell Exercises only)		Main Muscle Groups	Instructions
134	Every minute on the minute for 20 mins:			
	(1)	5 Jump Squats	Legs, Glutes, Core	Perform squat then jump, holding dumbbells.
	(2)	10 Bench Presses	Chest, Shoulders, Triceps	Press dumbbells from chest to straight arms on a bench.
	(3)	15 Russian Twists	Core, Obliques, Shoulders	Rotate torso holding dumbbell, seated with legs lifted.
135	5 Rounds for time:			
	(1)	10 Sumo Squats	Legs, Glutes, Core	Squat with wide stance, holding dumbbell.
	(2)	12 Seesaw Rows	Back, Biceps, Core	Row one dumbbell while other lowers, alternating.
	(3)	15 Plank Ts	Core, Shoulders, Arms	Rotate into T position from plank with dumbbell.
136	45 secs work / 15 secs rest per exercise for 4 rounds:			
	(1)	Dumbbell Swing	Legs, Core, Shoulders	Swing dumbbell between legs then up to shoulder height.
	(2)	Reverse Fly	Shoulders, Upper Back	Lift dumbbells outward while bent over.
	(3)	Calf Raise	Calves, Legs	Lift heels off the ground while holding dumbbells.
137	20 mins AMRAP (as many rounds as possible):			
	(1)	10 Alternating Front Raises	Shoulders, Core	Lift dumbbells to shoulder height, alternating arms.
	(2)	12 Glute Bridges	Glutes, Hamstrings, Core	Lift hips while holding dumbbell on hips.
	(3)	15 Concentration Curls	Biceps	Curl dumbbell with elbow on thigh, focus on bicep.
138	30 secs work / 30 secs rest per exercise for 5 rounds:			
	(1)	Farmer's Walk	Shoulders, Core, Legs	Walk holding heavy dumbbells at sides.
	(2)	Reverse Lunge	Legs, Glutes, Core	Step back into lunge, holding dumbbells at sides.
	(3)	Side Raise	Shoulders, Core	Lift dumbbells to sides, shoulder height.
139	4 Rounds for time:			
	(1)	10 Romanian Deadlifts	Hamstrings, Glutes, Lower Back	Lower dumbbells to shins with slight knee bend, then lift.
	(2)	12 Tricep Extensions	Triceps, Shoulders	Extend dumbbell overhead, bending elbow.
	(3)	15 Floor T Raises	Shoulders, Upper Back	Lift dumbbells to form T-shape while lying face down.
140	Every minute on the minute for 16 mins:			
	(1)	5 Goblet Squats	Legs, Glutes, Core	Hold dumbbell at chest, perform deep squat.
	(2)	10 Shoulder Presses	Shoulders, Triceps	Press dumbbells overhead from shoulders.
	(3)	15 Russian Twists	Core, Obliques, Shoulders	Rotate torso holding dumbbell, seated with legs lifted.

Workout No.	Workout (Dumbbell Exercises only)	Main Muscle Groups	Instructions
141	**5 Rounds for time:**		
	(1) 10 Thrusters	Shoulders, Legs, Core	Squat down, then press dumbbells overhead in one motion.
	(2) 15 Renegade Rows	Back, Shoulders, Core	Row dumbbell from plank position, alternating sides.
	(3) 20 Russian Twists	Core, Obliques, Shoulders	Rotate torso holding dumbbell, seated with legs lifted.
142	**As many rounds as possible in 12 mins of:**		
	(1) 10 Goblet Squats	Legs, Glutes, Core	Hold dumbbell at chest, perform deep squat.
	(2) 15 Single Arm Rows (each side)	Back, Biceps, Core	Row dumbbell to hip while bent over, switch sides.
	(3) 20 Hammer Curls	Biceps, Forearms	Curl dumbbells with palms facing each other.
143	**4 Rounds for time:**		
	(1) 12 Step-Ups (each leg)	Legs, Glutes, Core	Step onto platform holding dumbbells, alternating legs.
	(2) 15 Shoulder Presses	Shoulders, Triceps	Press dumbbells overhead from shoulders.
	(3) 20 V-Sit Cross Jabs	Core, Shoulders, Arms	Sit in V position, punch across body with dumbbell.
144	**Every minute on the minute for 20 mins:**		
	(1) 5 Jump Squats	Legs, Glutes, Core	Perform squat then jump, holding dumbbells.
	(2) 10 Bench Presses	Chest, Shoulders, Triceps	Press dumbbells from chest to straight arms on a bench.
	(3) 15 Russian Twists	Core, Obliques, Shoulders	Rotate torso holding dumbbell, seated with legs lifted.
145	**5 Rounds for time:**		
	(1) 10 Sumo Squats	Legs, Glutes, Core	Squat with wide stance, holding dumbbell.
	(2) 12 Seesaw Rows	Back, Biceps, Core	Row one dumbbell while other lowers, alternating.
	(3) 15 Plank Ts	Core, Shoulders, Arms	Rotate into T position from plank with dumbbell.
146	**45 secs work / 15 secs rest per exercise for 4 rounds:**		
	(1) Dumbbell Swing	Legs, Core, Shoulders	Swing dumbbell between legs then up to shoulder height.
	(2) Reverse Fly	Shoulders, Upper Back	Lift dumbbells outward while bent over.
	(3) Calf Raise	Calves, Legs	Lift heels off the ground while holding dumbbells.
147	**20 mins AMRAP (as many rounds as possible):**		
	(1) 10 Alternating Front Raises	Shoulders, Core	Lift dumbbells to shoulder height, alternating arms.
	(2) 12 Glute Bridges	Glutes, Hamstrings, Core	Lift hips while holding dumbbell on hips.
	(3) 15 Concentration Curls	Biceps	Curl dumbbell with elbow on thigh, focus on bicep.

Workout No.		Workout (Dumbbell Exercises only)	Main Muscle Groups	Instructions
148		**30 secs work / 30 secs rest per exercise for 5 rounds:**		
	(1)	Farmer's Walk	Shoulders, Core, Legs	Walk holding heavy dumbbells at sides.
	(2)	Reverse Lunge	Legs, Glutes, Core	Step back into lunge, holding dumbbells at sides.
	(3)	Side Raise	Shoulders, Core	Lift dumbbells to sides, shoulder height.
149		**4 Rounds for time:**		
	(1)	10 Romanian Deadlifts	Hamstrings, Glutes, Lower Back	Lower dumbbells to shins with slight knee bend, then lift.
	(2)	12 Tricep Extensions	Triceps, Shoulders	Extend dumbbell overhead, bending elbow.
	(3)	15 Floor T Raises	Shoulders, Upper Back	Lift dumbbells to form T-shape while lying face down.
150		**Every minute on the minute for 16 mins:**		
	(1)	5 Goblet Squats	Legs, Glutes, Core	Hold dumbbell at chest, perform deep squat.
	(2)	10 Shoulder Presses	Shoulders, Triceps	Press dumbbells overhead from shoulders.
	(3)	15 Russian Twists	Core, Obliques, Shoulders	Rotate torso holding dumbbell, seated with legs lifted.

Part II

150 Dumbbell + Body-Weight Workouts

Workout No.	Workout (Dumbbell and Body-Weight)	Main Muscle Groups	Instructions
1	**5 Rounds:**		
	(1) Jumping Jacks - 1 minute	Cardio, Legs, Shoulders	Jump feet out and clap hands overhead, return quickly. Maintain speed and light
	(2) Dumbbell Thrusters - 12 reps	Legs, Shoulders, Core	Squat down holding dumbbells at shoulders, explode up and press
	(3) Burpees - 1 minute	Full Body, Cardio, Core	Jump, drop into push-up position, perform push-up, jump back up.
2	**3 Rounds for time:**		
	(1) Dumbbell Deadlift - 15 reps	Back, Legs, Core	Lower dumbbells to shins with slight knee bend, then lift.
	(2) Push-Ups - 20 reps	Chest, Triceps, Core	Lower chest to ground, push back up. Keep body straight.
	(3) Dumbbell Step-Ups - 12 reps each leg	Legs, Glutes, Core	Step onto platform holding dumbbells, alternate legs.
3	**4 Rounds:**		
	(1) High Knees - 45 seconds	Cardio, Legs, Core	Run in place lifting knees high, maintain pace.
	(2) Dumbbell Shoulder Press - 15 reps	Shoulders, Triceps, Core	Press dumbbells overhead from shoulders, keep core tight.
	(3) V-Ups - 45 seconds	Abs, Core, Hip Flexors	Lie back, lift legs and torso simultaneously, form 'V'.
4	**As many rounds as possible in 15 mins of:**		
	(1) Dumbbell Snatch - 10 reps each arm	Shoulders, Back, Core	Lift dumbbell from floor to overhead in one movement, alternate arms.
	(2) Sit-Ups - 20 reps	Abs, Core, Hip Flexors	Lie back, sit up and touch toes. Control descent.
	(3) Dumbbell Lunges - 12 reps each leg	Legs, Glutes, Core	Step forward into lunge holding dumbbells, switch legs.
5	**5 Rounds:**		
	(1) Burpees - 30 seconds	Full Body, Cardio, Core	Jump, drop into push-up position, perform push-up, jump back up.
	(2) Dumbbell Rows - 15 reps each arm	Back, Biceps, Core	Row dumbbell to hip while bent over, switch sides.
	(3) Mountain Climbers - 30 seconds	Cardio, Core, Shoulders	Run in place in plank position, drive knees to chest.
6	**For time:**		
	(1) Dumbbell Clean and Press - 15 reps	Full Body, Shoulders, Core	Lift dumbbells to shoulders from floor, press overhead.
	(2) Hand-Release Push-Ups - 20 reps	Chest, Triceps, Core	Lower chest to ground, lift hands, push back up.
	(3) Dumbbell Side Lunges - 12 reps each leg	Legs, Glutes, Core	Step sideways into lunge holding dumbbells, switch sides.
7	**4 Rounds:**		
	(1) Jump Squats - 1 minute	Legs, Glutes, Cardio	Perform squat then jump, holding dumbbells. Land softly.
	(2) Renegade Rows - 12 reps each arm	Back, Shoulders, Core	Row dumbbell from plank position, switch sides.
	(3) Spider-Man Push-Ups - 1 minute	Chest, Core, Shoulders	Perform push-up, bring knee to elbow, switch sides.
8	**5 Rounds for time:**		
	(1) Dumbbell Deadlifts - 20 reps	Back, Legs, Core	Lower dumbbells to shins with slight knee bend, then lift.
	(2) Push Press - 15 reps	Shoulders, Triceps, Core	Press dumbbells overhead from shoulders, use leg drive.
	(3) Sit-Ups - 20 reps	Abs, Core, Hip Flexors	Lie back, sit up and touch toes. Control descent.

Workout No.		Workout (Dumbbell and Body-Weight)	Main Muscle Groups	Instructions
9		**6 Rounds:**		
	(1)	Tuck Jumps - 45 seconds	Legs, Cardio, Core	Jump high, tuck knees to chest mid-air. Land softly.
	(2)	Dumbbell Bench Press - 15 reps	Chest, Triceps, Shoulders	Press dumbbells from chest to straight arms on a bench.
	(3)	Plank T - 45 seconds	Core, Shoulders, Back	Rotate into T position from plank with dumbbell, switch sides.
10		**3 Rounds for time:**		
	(1)	Dumbbell Front Squats - 20 reps	Legs, Glutes, Core	Hold dumbbells at shoulders, perform deep squat.
	(2)	Diamond Push-Ups - 15 reps	Chest, Triceps, Core	Push-up with hands under shoulders, elbows tight.
	(3)	Russian Twists - 20 reps	Core, Obliques, Abs	Twist torso holding dumbbell, seated with legs lifted.
11		**For time:**		
	(1)	Dumbbell Deadlift - 15 reps	Back, Legs, Core	Lower dumbbells to shins with slight knee bend, then lift. Keep back straight.
	(2)	Push-Ups - 20 reps	Chest, Triceps, Core	Lower chest to ground, push back up. Keep body straight.
	(3)	Dumbbell Step-Ups - 12 reps each leg	Legs, Glutes, Core	Step onto platform holding dumbbells, alternate legs.
12		**5 Rounds:**		
	(1)	Jumping Jacks - 1 minute	Cardio, Legs, Shoulders	Jump feet out and clap hands overhead, return quickly. Maintain speed and light
	(2)	Dumbbell Thrusters - 12 reps	Legs, Shoulders, Core	Squat down holding dumbbells at shoulders, explode up and press
	(3)	Burpees - 1 minute	Full Body, Cardio, Core	Jump, drop into push-up position, perform push-up, jump back up.
13		**As many rounds as possible in 15 mins of:**		
	(1)	Dumbbell Snatch - 10 reps each arm	Shoulders, Back, Core	Lift dumbbell from floor to overhead in one movement, alternate arms.
	(2)	Sit-Ups - 20 reps	Abs, Core, Hip Flexors	Lie back, sit up and touch toes. Control descent.
	(3)	Dumbbell Lunges - 12 reps each leg	Legs, Glutes, Core	Step forward into lunge holding dumbbells, switch legs.
14		**4 Rounds:**		
	(1)	High Knees - 45 seconds	Cardio, Legs, Core	Run in place lifting knees high, maintain pace.
	(2)	Dumbbell Shoulder Press - 15 reps	Shoulders, Triceps, Core	Press dumbbells overhead from shoulders, keep core tight.
	(3)	V-Ups - 45 seconds	Abs, Core, Hip Flexors	Lie back, lift legs and torso simultaneously, form 'V'.
15		**For time:**		
	(1)	Dumbbell Clean and Press - 15 reps	Full Body, Shoulders, Core	Lift dumbbells to shoulders from floor, press overhead.
	(2)	Hand-Release Push-Ups - 20 reps	Chest, Triceps, Core	Lower chest to ground, lift hands, push back up.
	(3)	Dumbbell Side Lunges - 12 reps each leg	Legs, Glutes, Core	Step sideways into lunge holding dumbbells, switch sides.
16		**5 Rounds:**		
	(1)	Burpees - 30 seconds	Full Body, Cardio, Core	Jump, drop into push-up position, perform push-up, jump back up.
	(2)	Dumbbell Rows - 15 reps each arm	Back, Biceps, Core	Row dumbbell to hip while bent over, switch sides.
	(3)	Mountain Climbers - 30 seconds	Cardio, Core, Shoulders	Run in place in plank position, drive knees to chest.

Workout No.	Workout (Dumbbell and Body-Weight)	Main Muscle Groups	Instructions
17	**3 Rounds for time:**		
	(1) Dumbbell Front Squats - 20 reps	Legs, Glutes, Core	Hold dumbbells at shoulders, perform deep squat.
	(2) Diamond Push-Ups - 15 reps	Chest, Triceps, Core	Push-up with hands under shoulders, elbows tight.
	(3) Dumbbell Swings - 20 reps	Core, Shoulders, Back	Swing dumbbell between legs then up to shoulder height.
18	**4 Rounds:**		
	(1) Jump Squats - 1 minute	Legs, Glutes, Cardio	Perform squat then jump, holding dumbbells. Land softly.
	(2) Renegade Rows - 12 reps each arm	Back, Shoulders, Core	Row dumbbell from plank position, switch sides.
	(3) Spider-Man Push-Ups - 1 minute	Chest, Core, Shoulders	Perform push-up, bring knee to elbow, switch sides.
19	**For time:**		
	(1) Dumbbell Bench Press - 20 reps	Chest, Triceps, Shoulders	Press dumbbells from chest to straight arms on a bench.
	(2) Walking Lunges - 15 reps each leg	Legs, Glutes, Core	Step forward into lunge holding dumbbells, switch legs.
	(3) Dumbbell Thrusters - 15 reps	Legs, Shoulders, Core	Squat down holding dumbbells at shoulders, explode up and press
20	**6 Rounds:**		
	(1) Tuck Jumps - 45 seconds	Legs, Cardio, Core	Jump high, tuck knees to chest mid-air. Land softly.
	(2) Dumbbell Plank T - 12 reps each side	Core, Shoulders, Back	Rotate into T position from plank with dumbbell, switch sides.
	(3) Push-Ups - 30 seconds	Chest, Triceps, Core	Lower chest to ground, push back up. Keep body straight.
21	**For time:**		
	(1) Dumbbell Deadlift - 15 reps	Back, Legs, Core	Lower dumbbells to shins with slight knee bend, then lift. Keep back straight.
	(2) Push-Ups - 20 reps	Chest, Triceps, Core	Lower chest to ground, push back up. Keep body straight.
	(3) Dumbbell Step-Ups - 12 reps each leg	Legs, Glutes, Core	Step onto platform holding dumbbells, alternate legs.
22	**5 Rounds:**		
	(1) Jumping Jacks - 1 minute	Cardio, Legs, Shoulders	Jump feet out and clap hands overhead, return quickly. Maintain speed and light
	(2) Dumbbell Thrusters - 12 reps	Legs, Shoulders, Core	Squat down holding dumbbells at shoulders, explode up and press
	(3) Burpees - 1 minute	Full Body, Cardio, Core	Jump, drop into push-up position, perform push-up, jump back up.
23	**As many rounds as possible in 15 mins of:**		
	(1) Dumbbell Snatch - 10 reps each arm	Shoulders, Back, Core	Lift dumbbell from floor to overhead in one movement, alternate arms.
	(2) Sit-Ups - 20 reps	Abs, Core, Hip Flexors	Lie back, sit up and touch toes. Control descent.
	(3) Dumbbell Lunges - 12 reps each leg	Legs, Glutes, Core	Step forward into lunge holding dumbbells, switch legs.
24	**4 Rounds:**		
	(1) High Knees - 45 seconds	Cardio, Legs, Core	Run in place lifting knees high, maintain pace.
	(2) Dumbbell Shoulder Press - 15 reps	Shoulders, Triceps, Core	Press dumbbells overhead from shoulders, keep core tight.
	(3) V-Ups - 45 seconds	Abs, Core, Hip Flexors	Lie back, lift legs and torso simultaneously, form 'V'.

Workout No.	Workout (Dumbbell and Body-Weight)	Main Muscle Groups	Instructions
25	**For time:**		
	(1) Dumbbell Clean and Press - 15 reps	Full Body, Shoulders, Core	Lift dumbbells to shoulders from floor, press overhead.
	(2) Hand-Release Push-Ups - 20 reps	Chest, Triceps, Core	Lower chest to ground, lift hands, push back up.
	(3) Dumbbell Side Lunges - 12 reps each leg	Legs, Glutes, Core	Step sideways into lunge holding dumbbells, switch sides.
26	**5 Rounds:**		
	(1) Burpees - 30 seconds	Full Body, Cardio, Core	Jump, drop into push-up position, perform push-up, jump back up.
	(2) Dumbbell Rows - 15 reps each arm	Back, Biceps, Core	Row dumbbell to hip while bent over, switch sides.
	(3) Mountain Climbers - 30 seconds	Cardio, Core, Shoulders	Run in place in plank position, drive knees to chest.
27	**3 Rounds for time:**		
	(1) Dumbbell Front Squats - 20 reps	Legs, Glutes, Core	Hold dumbbells at shoulders, perform deep squat.
	(2) Diamond Push-Ups - 15 reps	Chest, Triceps, Core	Push-up with hands under shoulders, elbows tight.
	(3) Dumbbell Swings - 20 reps	Core, Shoulders, Back	Swing dumbbell between legs then up to shoulder height.
28	**4 Rounds:**		
	(1) Jump Squats - 1 minute	Legs, Glutes, Cardio	Perform squat then jump, holding dumbbells. Land softly.
	(2) Renegade Rows - 12 reps each arm	Back, Shoulders, Core	Row dumbbell from plank position, switch sides.
	(3) Spider-Man Push-Ups - 1 minute	Chest, Core, Shoulders	Perform push-up, bring knee to elbow, switch sides.
29	**For time:**		
	(1) Dumbbell Bench Press - 20 reps	Chest, Triceps, Shoulders	Press dumbbells from chest to straight arms on a bench.
	(2) Walking Lunges - 15 reps each leg	Legs, Glutes, Core	Step forward into lunge holding dumbbells, switch legs.
	(3) Dumbbell Thrusters - 15 reps	Legs, Shoulders, Core	Squat down holding dumbbells at shoulders, explode up and press
30	**6 Rounds:**		
	(1) Tuck Jumps - 45 seconds	Legs, Cardio, Core	Jump high, tuck knees to chest mid-air. Land softly.
	(2) Dumbbell Plank T - 12 reps each side	Core, Shoulders, Back	Rotate into T position from plank with dumbbell, switch sides.
	(3) Push-Ups - 30 seconds	Chest, Triceps, Core	Lower chest to ground, push back up. Keep body straight.
31	**For time:**		
	(1) Dumbbell Deadlift - 15 reps	Back, Legs, Core	Lower dumbbells to shins with slight knee bend, then lift. Keep back straight.
	(2) Push-Ups - 20 reps	Chest, Triceps, Core	Lower chest to ground, push back up. Keep body straight.
	(3) Dumbbell Step-Ups - 12 reps each leg	Legs, Glutes, Core	Step onto platform holding dumbbells, alternate legs.
32	**5 Rounds:**		
	(1) Jumping Jacks - 1 minute	Cardio, Legs, Shoulders	Jump feet out and clap hands overhead, return quickly. Maintain speed and light
	(2) Dumbbell Thrusters - 12 reps	Legs, Shoulders, Core	Squat down holding dumbbells at shoulders, explode up and press
	(3) Burpees - 1 minute	Full Body, Cardio, Core	Jump, drop into push-up position, perform push-up, jump back up.

Workout No.	Workout (Dumbbell and Body-Weight)	Main Muscle Groups	Instructions
33	**As many rounds as possible in 15 mins of:**		
	(1) Dumbbell Snatch - 10 reps each arm	Shoulders, Back, Core	Lift dumbbell from floor to overhead in one movement, alternate arms.
	(2) Sit-Ups - 20 reps	Abs, Core, Hip Flexors	Lie back, sit up and touch toes. Control descent.
	(3) Dumbbell Lunges - 12 reps each leg	Legs, Glutes, Core	Step forward into lunge holding dumbbells, switch legs.
34	**4 Rounds:**		
	(1) High Knees - 45 seconds	Cardio, Legs, Core	Run in place lifting knees high, maintain pace.
	(2) Dumbbell Shoulder Press - 15 reps	Shoulders, Triceps, Core	Press dumbbells overhead from shoulders, keep core tight.
	(3) V-Ups - 45 seconds	Abs, Core, Hip Flexors	Lie back, lift legs and torso simultaneously, form 'V'.
35	**For time:**		
	(1) Dumbbell Clean and Press - 15 reps	Full Body, Shoulders, Core	Lift dumbbells to shoulders from floor, press overhead.
	(2) Hand-Release Push-Ups - 20 reps	Chest, Triceps, Core	Lower chest to ground, lift hands, push back up.
	(3) Dumbbell Side Lunges - 12 reps each leg	Legs, Glutes, Core	Step sideways into lunge holding dumbbells, switch sides.
36	**5 Rounds:**		
	(1) Burpees - 30 seconds	Full Body, Cardio, Core	Jump, drop into push-up position, perform push-up, jump back up.
	(2) Dumbbell Rows - 15 reps each arm	Back, Biceps, Core	Row dumbbell to hip while bent over, switch sides.
	(3) Mountain Climbers - 30 seconds	Cardio, Core, Shoulders	Run in place in plank position, drive knees to chest.
37	**3 Rounds for time:**		
	(1) Dumbbell Front Squats - 20 reps	Legs, Glutes, Core	Hold dumbbells at shoulders, perform deep squat.
	(2) Diamond Push-Ups - 15 reps	Chest, Triceps, Core	Push-up with hands under shoulders, elbows tight.
	(3) Dumbbell Swings - 20 reps	Core, Shoulders, Back	Swing dumbbell between legs then up to shoulder height.
38	**4 Rounds:**		
	(1) Jump Squats - 1 minute	Legs, Glutes, Cardio	Perform squat then jump, holding dumbbells. Land softly.
	(2) Renegade Rows - 12 reps each arm	Back, Shoulders, Core	Row dumbbell from plank position, switch sides.
	(3) Spider-Man Push-Ups - 1 minute	Chest, Core, Shoulders	Perform push-up, bring knee to elbow, switch sides.
39	**For time:**		
	(1) Dumbbell Bench Press - 20 reps	Chest, Triceps, Shoulders	Press dumbbells from chest to straight arms on a bench.
	(2) Walking Lunges - 15 reps each leg	Legs, Glutes, Core	Step forward into lunge holding dumbbells, switch legs.
	(3) Dumbbell Thrusters - 15 reps	Legs, Shoulders, Core	Squat down holding dumbbells at shoulders, explode up and press
40	**6 Rounds:**		
	(1) Tuck Jumps - 45 seconds	Legs, Cardio, Core	Jump high, tuck knees to chest mid-air. Land softly.
	(2) Dumbbell Plank T - 12 reps each side	Core, Shoulders, Back	Rotate into T position from plank with dumbbell, switch sides.
	(3) Push-Ups - 30 seconds	Chest, Triceps, Core	Lower chest to ground, push back up. Keep body straight.

Workout No.	Workout (Dumbbell and Body-Weight)		Main Muscle Groups	Instructions
41	**For time:**			
	(1)	Dumbbell Deadlift - 15 reps	Back, Legs, Core	Lower dumbbells to shins with slight knee bend, then lift. Keep back straight.
	(2)	Push-Ups - 20 reps	Chest, Triceps, Core	Lower chest to ground, push back up. Keep body straight.
	(3)	Dumbbell Step-Ups - 12 reps each leg	Legs, Glutes, Core	Step onto platform holding dumbbells, alternate legs.
42	**5 Rounds:**			
	(1)	Jumping Jacks - 1 minute	Cardio, Legs, Shoulders	Jump feet out and clap hands overhead, return quickly. Maintain speed and light
	(2)	Dumbbell Thrusters - 12 reps	Legs, Shoulders, Core	Squat down holding dumbbells at shoulders, explode up and press
	(3)	Burpees - 1 minute	Full Body, Cardio, Core	Jump, drop into push-up position, perform push-up, jump back up.
43	**As many rounds as possible in 15 mins of:**			
	(1)	Dumbbell Snatch - 10 reps each arm	Shoulders, Back, Core	Lift dumbbell from floor to overhead in one movement, alternate arms.
	(2)	Sit-Ups - 20 reps	Abs, Core, Hip Flexors	Lie back, sit up and touch toes. Control descent.
	(3)	Dumbbell Lunges - 12 reps each leg	Legs, Glutes, Core	Step forward into lunge holding dumbbells, switch legs.
44	**4 Rounds:**			
	(1)	High Knees - 45 seconds	Cardio, Legs, Core	Run in place lifting knees high, maintain pace.
	(2)	Dumbbell Shoulder Press - 15 reps	Shoulders, Triceps, Core	Press dumbbells overhead from shoulders, keep core tight.
	(3)	V-Ups - 45 seconds	Abs, Core, Hip Flexors	Lie back, lift legs and torso simultaneously, form 'V'.
45	**For time:**			
	(1)	Dumbbell Clean and Press - 15 reps	Full Body, Shoulders, Core	Lift dumbbells to shoulders from floor, press overhead.
	(2)	Hand-Release Push-Ups - 20 reps	Chest, Triceps, Core	Lower chest to ground, lift hands, push back up.
	(3)	Dumbbell Side Lunges - 12 reps each leg	Legs, Glutes, Core	Step sideways into lunge holding dumbbells, switch sides.
46	**5 Rounds:**			
	(1)	Burpees - 30 seconds	Full Body, Cardio, Core	Jump, drop into push-up position, perform push-up, jump back up.
	(2)	Dumbbell Rows - 15 reps each arm	Back, Biceps, Core	Row dumbbell to hip while bent over, switch sides.
	(3)	Mountain Climbers - 30 seconds	Cardio, Core, Shoulders	Run in place in plank position, drive knees to chest.
47	**3 Rounds for time:**			
	(1)	Dumbbell Front Squats - 20 reps	Legs, Glutes, Core	Hold dumbbells at shoulders, perform deep squat.
	(2)	Diamond Push-Ups - 15 reps	Chest, Triceps, Core	Push-up with hands under shoulders, elbows tight.
	(3)	Dumbbell Swings - 20 reps	Core, Shoulders, Back	Swing dumbbell between legs then up to shoulder height.
48	**4 Rounds:**			
	(1)	Jump Squats - 1 minute	Legs, Glutes, Cardio	Perform squat then jump, holding dumbbells. Land softly.
	(2)	Renegade Rows - 12 reps each arm	Back, Shoulders, Core	Row dumbbell from plank position, switch sides.
	(3)	Spider-Man Push-Ups - 1 minute	Chest, Core, Shoulders	Perform push-up, bring knee to elbow, switch sides.

Workout No.	Workout (Dumbbell and Body-Weight)	Main Muscle Groups	Instructions
49	**For time:**		
	(1) Dumbbell Bench Press - 20 reps	Chest, Triceps, Shoulders	Press dumbbells from chest to straight arms on a bench.
	(2) Walking Lunges - 15 reps each leg	Legs, Glutes, Core	Step forward into lunge holding dumbbells, switch legs.
	(3) Dumbbell Thrusters - 15 reps	Legs, Shoulders, Core	Squat down holding dumbbells at shoulders, explode up and press
50	**6 Rounds:**		
	(1) Tuck Jumps - 45 seconds	Legs, Cardio, Core	Jump high, tuck knees to chest mid-air. Land softly.
	(2) Dumbbell Plank T - 12 reps each side	Core, Shoulders, Back	Rotate into T position from plank with dumbbell, switch sides.
	(3) Push-Ups - 30 seconds	Chest, Triceps, Core	Lower chest to ground, push back up. Keep body straight.
51	**For time:**		
	(1) Dumbbell Deadlift - 15 reps	Back, Legs, Core	Lower dumbbells to shins with slight knee bend, then lift. Keep back straight.
	(2) Push-Ups - 20 reps	Chest, Triceps, Core	Lower chest to ground, push back up. Keep body straight.
	(3) Dumbbell Step-Ups - 12 reps each leg	Legs, Glutes, Core	Step onto platform holding dumbbells, alternate legs.
52	**5 Rounds:**		
	(1) Jumping Jacks - 1 minute	Cardio, Legs, Shoulders	Jump feet out and clap hands overhead, return quickly. Maintain speed and light
	(2) Dumbbell Thrusters - 12 reps	Legs, Shoulders, Core	Squat down holding dumbbells at shoulders, explode up and press
	(3) Burpees - 1 minute	Full Body, Cardio, Core	Jump, drop into push-up position, perform push-up, jump back up.
53	**As many rounds as possible in 15 mins of:**		
	(1) Dumbbell Snatch - 10 reps each arm	Shoulders, Back, Core	Lift dumbbell from floor to overhead in one movement, alternate arms.
	(2) Sit-Ups - 20 reps	Abs, Core, Hip Flexors	Lie back, sit up and touch toes. Control descent.
	(3) Dumbbell Lunges - 12 reps each leg	Legs, Glutes, Core	Step forward into lunge holding dumbbells, switch legs.
54	**4 Rounds:**		
	(1) High Knees - 45 seconds	Cardio, Legs, Core	Run in place lifting knees high, maintain pace.
	(2) Dumbbell Shoulder Press - 15 reps	Shoulders, Triceps, Core	Press dumbbells overhead from shoulders, keep core tight.
	(3) V-Ups - 45 seconds	Abs, Core, Hip Flexors	Lie back, lift legs and torso simultaneously, form 'V'.
55	**For time:**		
	(1) Dumbbell Clean and Press - 15 reps	Full Body, Shoulders, Core	Lift dumbbells to shoulders from floor, press overhead.
	(2) Hand-Release Push-Ups - 20 reps	Chest, Triceps, Core	Lower chest to ground, lift hands, push back up.
	(3) Dumbbell Side Lunges - 12 reps each leg	Legs, Glutes, Core	Step sideways into lunge holding dumbbells, switch sides.
56	**5 Rounds:**		
	(1) Burpees - 30 seconds	Full Body, Cardio, Core	Jump, drop into push-up position, perform push-up, jump back up.
	(2) Dumbbell Rows - 15 reps each arm	Back, Biceps, Core	Row dumbbell to hip while bent over, switch sides.
	(3) Mountain Climbers - 30 seconds	Cardio, Core, Shoulders	Run in place in plank position, drive knees to chest.

Workout No.	Workout (Dumbbell and Body-Weight)		Main Muscle Groups	Instructions
57	**3 Rounds for time:**			
	(1)	Dumbbell Front Squats - 20 reps	Legs, Glutes, Core	Hold dumbbells at shoulders, perform deep squat.
	(2)	Diamond Push-Ups - 15 reps	Chest, Triceps, Core	Push-up with hands under shoulders, elbows tight.
	(3)	Dumbbell Swings - 20 reps	Core, Shoulders, Back	Swing dumbbell between legs then up to shoulder height.
58	**4 Rounds:**			
	(1)	Jump Squats - 1 minute	Legs, Glutes, Cardio	Perform squat then jump, holding dumbbells. Land softly.
	(2)	Renegade Rows - 12 reps each arm	Back, Shoulders, Core	Row dumbbell from plank position, switch sides.
	(3)	Spider-Man Push-Ups - 1 minute	Chest, Core, Shoulders	Perform push-up, bring knee to elbow, switch sides.
59	**For time:**			
	(1)	Dumbbell Bench Press - 20 reps	Chest, Triceps, Shoulders	Press dumbbells from chest to straight arms on a bench.
	(2)	Walking Lunges - 15 reps each leg	Legs, Glutes, Core	Step forward into lunge holding dumbbells, switch legs.
	(3)	Dumbbell Thrusters - 15 reps	Legs, Shoulders, Core	Squat down holding dumbbells at shoulders, explode up and press
60	**6 Rounds:**			
	(1)	Tuck Jumps - 45 seconds	Legs, Cardio, Core	Jump high, tuck knees to chest mid-air. Land softly.
	(2)	Dumbbell Plank T - 12 reps each side	Core, Shoulders, Back	Rotate into T position from plank with dumbbell, switch sides.
	(3)	Push-Ups - 30 seconds	Chest, Triceps, Core	Lower chest to ground, push back up. Keep body straight.
61	**For time:**			
	(1)	Dumbbell Deadlift - 15 reps	Back, Legs, Core	Lower dumbbells to shins with slight knee bend, then lift. Keep back straight.
	(2)	Push-Ups - 20 reps	Chest, Triceps, Core	Lower chest to ground, push back up. Keep body straight.
	(3)	Dumbbell Step-Ups - 12 reps each leg	Legs, Glutes, Core	Step onto platform holding dumbbells, alternate legs.
62	**5 Rounds:**			
	(1)	Jumping Jacks - 1 minute	Cardio, Legs, Shoulders	Jump feet out and clap hands overhead, return quickly. Maintain speed and light
	(2)	Dumbbell Thrusters - 12 reps	Legs, Shoulders, Core	Squat down holding dumbbells at shoulders, explode up and press
	(3)	Burpees - 1 minute	Full Body, Cardio, Core	Jump, drop into push-up position, perform push-up, jump back up.
63	**As many rounds as possible in 15 mins of:**			
	(1)	Dumbbell Snatch - 10 reps each arm	Shoulders, Back, Core	Lift dumbbell from floor to overhead in one movement, alternate arms.
	(2)	Sit-Ups - 20 reps	Abs, Core, Hip Flexors	Lie back, sit up and touch toes. Control descent.
	(3)	Dumbbell Lunges - 12 reps each leg	Legs, Glutes, Core	Step forward into lunge holding dumbbells, switch legs.
64	**4 Rounds:**			
	(1)	High Knees - 45 seconds	Cardio, Legs, Core	Run in place lifting knees high, maintain pace.
	(2)	Dumbbell Shoulder Press - 15 reps	Shoulders, Triceps, Core	Press dumbbells overhead from shoulders, keep core tight.
	(3)	V-Ups - 45 seconds	Abs, Core, Hip Flexors	Lie back, lift legs and torso simultaneously, form 'V'.

Workout No.	Workout (Dumbbell and Body-Weight)	Main Muscle Groups	Instructions
65	**For time:**		
	(1) Dumbbell Clean and Press - 15 reps	Full Body, Shoulders, Core	Lift dumbbells to shoulders from floor, press overhead.
	(2) Hand-Release Push-Ups - 20 reps	Chest, Triceps, Core	Lower chest to ground, lift hands, push back up.
	(3) Dumbbell Side Lunges - 12 reps each leg	Legs, Glutes, Core	Step sideways into lunge holding dumbbells, switch sides.
66	**5 Rounds:**		
	(1) Burpees - 30 seconds	Full Body, Cardio, Core	Jump, drop into push-up position, perform push-up, jump back up.
	(2) Dumbbell Rows - 15 reps each arm	Back, Biceps, Core	Row dumbbell to hip while bent over, switch sides.
	(3) Mountain Climbers - 30 seconds	Cardio, Core, Shoulders	Run in place in plank position, drive knees to chest.
67	**3 Rounds for time:**		
	(1) Dumbbell Front Squats - 20 reps	Legs, Glutes, Core	Hold dumbbells at shoulders, perform deep squat.
	(2) Diamond Push-Ups - 15 reps	Chest, Triceps, Core	Push-up with hands under shoulders, elbows tight.
	(3) Dumbbell Swings - 20 reps	Core, Shoulders, Back	Swing dumbbell between legs then up to shoulder height.
68	**4 Rounds:**		
	(1) Jump Squats - 1 minute	Legs, Glutes, Cardio	Perform squat then jump, holding dumbbells. Land softly.
	(2) Renegade Rows - 12 reps each arm	Back, Shoulders, Core	Row dumbbell from plank position, switch sides.
	(3) Spider-Man Push-Ups - 1 minute	Chest, Core, Shoulders	Perform push-up, bring knee to elbow, switch sides.
69	**For time:**		
	(1) Dumbbell Bench Press - 20 reps	Chest, Triceps, Shoulders	Press dumbbells from chest to straight arms on a bench.
	(2) Walking Lunges - 15 reps each leg	Legs, Glutes, Core	Step forward into lunge holding dumbbells, switch legs.
	(3) Dumbbell Thrusters - 15 reps	Legs, Shoulders, Core	Squat down holding dumbbells at shoulders, explode up and press
70	**6 Rounds:**		
	(1) Tuck Jumps - 45 seconds	Legs, Cardio, Core	Jump high, tuck knees to chest mid-air. Land softly.
	(2) Dumbbell Plank T - 12 reps each side	Core, Shoulders, Back	Rotate into T position from plank with dumbbell, switch sides.
	(3) Push-Ups - 30 seconds	Chest, Triceps, Core	Lower chest to ground, push back up. Keep body straight.
71	**For time:**		
	(1) Dumbbell Deadlift - 15 reps	Back, Legs, Core	Lower dumbbells to shins with slight knee bend, then lift. Keep back straight.
	(2) Push-Ups - 20 reps	Chest, Triceps, Core	Lower chest to ground, push back up. Keep body straight.
	(3) Dumbbell Step-Ups - 12 reps each leg	Legs, Glutes, Core	Step onto platform holding dumbbells, alternate legs.
72	**5 Rounds:**		
	(1) Jumping Jacks - 1 minute	Cardio, Legs, Shoulders	Jump feet out and clap hands overhead, return quickly. Maintain speed and light
	(2) Dumbbell Thrusters - 12 reps	Legs, Shoulders, Core	Squat down holding dumbbells at shoulders, explode up and press
	(3) Burpees - 1 minute	Full Body, Cardio, Core	Jump, drop into push-up position, perform push-up, jump back up.

Workout No.		Workout (Dumbbell and Body-Weight)	Main Muscle Groups	Instructions
73		**As many rounds as possible in 15 mins of:**		
	(1)	Dumbbell Snatch - 10 reps each arm	Shoulders, Back, Core	Lift dumbbell from floor to overhead in one movement, alternate arms.
	(2)	Sit-Ups - 20 reps	Abs, Core, Hip Flexors	Lie back, sit up and touch toes. Control descent.
	(3)	Dumbbell Lunges - 12 reps each leg	Legs, Glutes, Core	Step forward into lunge holding dumbbells, switch legs.
74		**4 Rounds:**		
	(1)	High Knees - 45 seconds	Cardio, Legs, Core	Run in place lifting knees high, maintain pace.
	(2)	Dumbbell Shoulder Press - 15 reps	Shoulders, Triceps, Core	Press dumbbells overhead from shoulders, keep core tight.
	(3)	V-Ups - 45 seconds	Abs, Core, Hip Flexors	Lie back, lift legs and torso simultaneously, form 'V'.
75		**For time:**		
	(1)	Dumbbell Clean and Press - 15 reps	Full Body, Shoulders, Core	Lift dumbbells to shoulders from floor, press overhead.
	(2)	Hand-Release Push-Ups - 20 reps	Chest, Triceps, Core	Lower chest to ground, lift hands, push back up.
	(3)	Dumbbell Side Lunges - 12 reps each leg	Legs, Glutes, Core	Step sideways into lunge holding dumbbells, switch sides.
76		**5 Rounds:**		
	(1)	Burpees - 30 seconds	Full Body, Cardio, Core	Jump, drop into push-up position, perform push-up, jump back up.
	(2)	Dumbbell Rows - 15 reps each arm	Back, Biceps, Core	Row dumbbell to hip while bent over, switch sides.
	(3)	Mountain Climbers - 30 seconds	Cardio, Core, Shoulders	Run in place in plank position, drive knees to chest.
77		**3 Rounds for time:**		
	(1)	Dumbbell Front Squats - 20 reps	Legs, Glutes, Core	Hold dumbbells at shoulders, perform deep squat.
	(2)	Diamond Push-Ups - 15 reps	Chest, Triceps, Core	Push-up with hands under shoulders, elbows tight.
	(3)	Dumbbell Swings - 20 reps	Core, Shoulders, Back	Swing dumbbell between legs then up to shoulder height.
78		**4 Rounds:**		
	(1)	Jump Squats - 1 minute	Legs, Glutes, Cardio	Perform squat then jump, holding dumbbells. Land softly.
	(2)	Renegade Rows - 12 reps each arm	Back, Shoulders, Core	Row dumbbell from plank position, switch sides.
	(3)	Spider-Man Push-Ups - 1 minute	Chest, Core, Shoulders	Perform push-up, bring knee to elbow, switch sides.
79		**For time:**		
	(1)	Dumbbell Bench Press - 20 reps	Chest, Triceps, Shoulders	Press dumbbells from chest to straight arms on a bench.
	(2)	Walking Lunges - 15 reps each leg	Legs, Glutes, Core	Step forward into lunge holding dumbbells, switch legs.
	(3)	Dumbbell Thrusters - 15 reps	Legs, Shoulders, Core	Squat down holding dumbbells at shoulders, explode up and press
80		**6 Rounds:**		
	(1)	Tuck Jumps - 45 seconds	Legs, Cardio, Core	Jump high, tuck knees to chest mid-air. Land softly.
	(2)	Dumbbell Plank T - 12 reps each side	Core, Shoulders, Back	Rotate into T position from plank with dumbbell, switch sides.
	(3)	Push-Ups - 30 seconds	Chest, Triceps, Core	Lower chest to ground, push back up. Keep body straight.

Workout No.	Workout (Dumbbell and Body-Weight)	Main Muscle Groups	Instructions
81	**As many rounds as possible in 15 mins of:**		
	(1) Dumbbell Deadlift - 15 reps	Back, Legs, Core	Lower dumbbells to shins with slight knee bend, then lift. Keep back straight.
	(2) Push-Ups - 20 reps	Chest, Triceps, Core	Lower chest to ground, push back up. Keep body straight.
	(3) Dumbbell Step-Ups - 12 reps each leg	Legs, Glutes, Core	Step onto platform holding dumbbells, alternate legs.
82	**5 Rounds:**		
	(1) Jumping Jacks - 1 minute	Cardio, Legs, Shoulders	Jump feet out and clap hands overhead, return quickly. Maintain speed and light
	(2) Dumbbell Thrusters - 12 reps	Legs, Shoulders, Core	Squat down holding dumbbells at shoulders, explode up and press
	(3) Burpees - 1 minute	Full Body, Cardio, Core	Jump, drop into push-up position, perform push-up, jump back up.
83	**As many rounds as possible in 12 mins of:**		
	(1) Dumbbell Snatch - 10 reps each arm	Shoulders, Back, Core	Lift dumbbell from floor to overhead in one movement, alternate arms.
	(2) Sit-Ups - 20 reps	Abs, Core, Hip Flexors	Lie back, sit up and touch toes. Control descent.
	(3) Dumbbell Lunges - 12 reps each leg	Legs, Glutes, Core	Step forward into lunge holding dumbbells, switch legs.
84	**4 Rounds:**		
	(1) High Knees - 45 seconds	Cardio, Legs, Core	Run in place lifting knees high, maintain pace.
	(2) Dumbbell Shoulder Press - 15 reps	Shoulders, Triceps, Core	Press dumbbells overhead from shoulders, keep core tight.
	(3) V-Ups - 45 seconds	Abs, Core, Hip Flexors	Lie back, lift legs and torso simultaneously, form 'V'.
85	**For time:**		
	(1) Dumbbell Clean and Press - 15 reps	Full Body, Shoulders, Core	Lift dumbbells to shoulders from floor, press overhead.
	(2) Hand-Release Push-Ups - 20 reps	Chest, Triceps, Core	Lower chest to ground, lift hands, push back up.
	(3) Dumbbell Side Lunges - 12 reps each leg	Legs, Glutes, Core	Step sideways into lunge holding dumbbells, switch sides.
86	**5 Rounds:**		
	(1) Burpees - 30 seconds	Full Body, Cardio, Core	Jump, drop into push-up position, perform push-up, jump back up.
	(2) Dumbbell Rows - 15 reps each arm	Back, Biceps, Core	Row dumbbell to hip while bent over, switch sides.
	(3) Mountain Climbers - 30 seconds	Cardio, Core, Shoulders	Run in place in plank position, drive knees to chest.
87	**3 Rounds for time:**		
	(1) Dumbbell Front Squats - 20 reps	Legs, Glutes, Core	Hold dumbbells at shoulders, perform deep squat.
	(2) Diamond Push-Ups - 15 reps	Chest, Triceps, Core	Push-up with hands under shoulders, elbows tight.
	(3) Dumbbell Swings - 20 reps	Core, Shoulders, Back	Swing dumbbell between legs then up to shoulder height.
88	**4 Rounds:**		
	(1) Jump Squats - 1 minute	Legs, Glutes, Cardio	Perform squat then jump, holding dumbbells. Land softly.
	(2) Renegade Rows - 12 reps each arm	Back, Shoulders, Core	Row dumbbell from plank position, switch sides.
	(3) Spider-Man Push-Ups - 1 minute	Chest, Core, Shoulders	Perform push-up, bring knee to elbow, switch sides.

Workout No.		Workout (Dumbbell and Body-Weight)	Main Muscle Groups	Instructions
89		**For time:**		
	(1)	Dumbbell Bench Press - 20 reps	Chest, Triceps, Shoulders	Press dumbbells from chest to straight arms on a bench.
	(2)	Walking Lunges - 15 reps each leg	Legs, Glutes, Core	Step forward into lunge holding dumbbells, switch legs.
	(3)	Dumbbell Thrusters - 15 reps	Legs, Shoulders, Core	Squat down holding dumbbells at shoulders, explode up and press
90		**6 Rounds:**		
	(1)	Tuck Jumps - 45 seconds	Legs, Cardio, Core	Jump high, tuck knees to chest mid-air. Land softly.
	(2)	Dumbbell Plank T - 12 reps each side	Core, Shoulders, Back	Rotate into T position from plank with dumbbell, switch sides.
	(3)	Push-Ups - 30 seconds	Chest, Triceps, Core	Lower chest to ground, push back up. Keep body straight.
91		**As many rounds as possible in 15 mins of:**		
	(1)	Dumbbell Deadlift - 15 reps	Back, Legs, Core	Lower dumbbells to shins with slight knee bend, then lift. Keep back straight.
	(2)	Push-Ups - 20 reps	Chest, Triceps, Core	Lower chest to ground, push back up. Keep body straight.
	(3)	Dumbbell Step-Ups - 12 reps each leg	Legs, Glutes, Core	Step onto platform holding dumbbells, alternate legs.
92		**5 Rounds:**		
	(1)	Jumping Jacks - 1 minute	Cardio, Legs, Shoulders	Jump feet out and clap hands overhead, return quickly. Maintain speed and light
	(2)	Dumbbell Thrusters - 12 reps	Legs, Shoulders, Core	Squat down holding dumbbells at shoulders, explode up and press
	(3)	Burpees - 1 minute	Full Body, Cardio, Core	Jump, drop into push-up position, perform push-up, jump back up.
93		**As many rounds as possible in 12 mins of:**		
	(1)	Dumbbell Snatch - 10 reps each arm	Shoulders, Back, Core	Lift dumbbell from floor to overhead in one movement, alternate arms.
	(2)	Sit-Ups - 20 reps	Abs, Core, Hip Flexors	Lie back, sit up and touch toes. Control descent.
	(3)	Dumbbell Lunges - 12 reps each leg	Legs, Glutes, Core	Step forward into lunge holding dumbbells, switch legs.
94		**4 Rounds:**		
	(1)	High Knees - 45 seconds	Cardio, Legs, Core	Run in place lifting knees high, maintain pace.
	(2)	Dumbbell Shoulder Press - 15 reps	Shoulders, Triceps, Core	Press dumbbells overhead from shoulders, keep core tight.
	(3)	V-Ups - 45 seconds	Abs, Core, Hip Flexors	Lie back, lift legs and torso simultaneously, form 'V'.
95		**For time:**		
	(1)	Dumbbell Clean and Press - 15 reps	Full Body, Shoulders, Core	Lift dumbbells to shoulders from floor, press overhead.
	(2)	Hand-Release Push-Ups - 20 reps	Chest, Triceps, Core	Lower chest to ground, lift hands, push back up.
	(3)	Dumbbell Side Lunges - 12 reps each leg	Legs, Glutes, Core	Step sideways into lunge holding dumbbells, switch sides.
96		**5 Rounds:**		
	(1)	Burpees - 30 seconds	Full Body, Cardio, Core	Jump, drop into push-up position, perform push-up, jump back up.
	(2)	Dumbbell Rows - 15 reps each arm	Back, Biceps, Core	Row dumbbell to hip while bent over, switch sides.
	(3)	Mountain Climbers - 30 seconds	Cardio, Core, Shoulders	Run in place in plank position, drive knees to chest.

Workout No.	Workout (Dumbbell and Body-Weight)	Main Muscle Groups	Instructions
97	**3 Rounds for time:**		
	(1) Dumbbell Front Squats - 20 reps	Legs, Glutes, Core	Hold dumbbells at shoulders, perform deep squat.
	(2) Diamond Push-Ups - 15 reps	Chest, Triceps, Core	Push-up with hands under shoulders, elbows tight.
	(3) Dumbbell Swings - 20 reps	Core, Shoulders, Back	Swing dumbbell between legs then up to shoulder height.
98	**4 Rounds:**		
	(1) Jump Squats - 1 minute	Legs, Glutes, Cardio	Perform squat then jump, holding dumbbells. Land softly.
	(2) Renegade Rows - 12 reps each arm	Back, Shoulders, Core	Row dumbbell from plank position, switch sides.
	(3) Spider-Man Push-Ups - 1 minute	Chest, Core, Shoulders	Perform push-up, bring knee to elbow, switch sides.
99	**For time:**		
	(1) Dumbbell Bench Press - 20 reps	Chest, Triceps, Shoulders	Press dumbbells from chest to straight arms on a bench.
	(2) Walking Lunges - 15 reps each leg	Legs, Glutes, Core	Step forward into lunge holding dumbbells, switch legs.
	(3) Dumbbell Thrusters - 15 reps	Legs, Shoulders, Core	Squat down holding dumbbells at shoulders, explode up and press
100	**6 Rounds:**		
	(1) Tuck Jumps - 45 seconds	Legs, Cardio, Core	Jump high, tuck knees to chest mid-air. Land softly.
	(2) Dumbbell Plank T - 12 reps each side	Core, Shoulders, Back	Rotate into T position from plank with dumbbell, switch sides.
	(3) Push-Ups - 30 seconds	Chest, Triceps, Core	Lower chest to ground, push back up. Keep body straight.
101	**For time:**		
	(1) Dumbbell Deadlift - 15 reps	Back, Legs, Core	Lower dumbbells to shins with slight knee bend, then lift. Keep back straight.
	(2) Push-Ups - 20 reps	Chest, Triceps, Core	Lower chest to ground, push back up. Keep body straight.
	(3) Dumbbell Step-Ups - 12 reps each leg	Legs, Glutes, Core	Step onto platform holding dumbbells, alternate legs.
	(4) Sit-Ups - 20 reps	Abs, Core, Hip Flexors	Lie back, sit up and touch toes. Control descent.
102	**5 Rounds:**		
	(1) Jumping Jacks - 1 minute	Cardio, Legs, Shoulders	Jump feet out and clap hands overhead, return quickly. Maintain speed and light
	(2) Dumbbell Thrusters - 12 reps	Legs, Shoulders, Core	Squat down holding dumbbells at shoulders, explode up and press
	(3) Burpees - 1 minute	Full Body, Cardio, Core	Jump, drop into push-up position, perform push-up, jump back up.
103	**As many rounds as possible in 12 mins of:**		
	(1) Dumbbell Snatch - 10 reps each arm	Shoulders, Back, Core	Lift dumbbell from floor to overhead in one movement, alternate arms.
	(2) Sit-Ups - 20 reps	Abs, Core, Hip Flexors	Lie back, sit up and touch toes. Control descent.
	(3) Dumbbell Lunges - 12 reps each leg	Legs, Glutes, Core	Step forward into lunge holding dumbbells, switch legs.
104	**4 Rounds:**		
	(1) High Knees - 45 seconds	Cardio, Legs, Core	Run in place lifting knees high, maintain pace.
	(2) Dumbbell Shoulder Press - 15 reps	Shoulders, Triceps, Core	Press dumbbells overhead from shoulders, keep core tight.
	(3) V-Ups - 45 seconds	Abs, Core, Hip Flexors	Lie back, lift legs and torso simultaneously, form 'V'.

Workout No.	Workout (Dumbbell and Body-Weight)	Main Muscle Groups	Instructions
105	**For time:**		
	(1) Dumbbell Clean and Press - 15 reps	Full Body, Shoulders, Core	Lift dumbbells to shoulders from floor, press overhead.
	(2) Hand-Release Push-Ups - 20 reps	Chest, Triceps, Core	Lower chest to ground, lift hands, push back up.
	(3) Dumbbell Side Lunges - 12 reps each leg	Legs, Glutes, Core	Step sideways into lunge holding dumbbells, switch sides.
106	**5 Rounds:**		
	(1) Burpees - 30 seconds	Full Body, Cardio, Core	Jump, drop into push-up position, perform push-up, jump back up.
	(2) Dumbbell Rows - 15 reps each arm	Back, Biceps, Core	Row dumbbell to hip while bent over, switch sides.
	(3) Mountain Climbers - 30 seconds	Cardio, Core, Shoulders	Run in place in plank position, drive knees to chest.
107	**3 Rounds for time:**		
	(1) Dumbbell Front Squats - 20 reps	Legs, Glutes, Core	Hold dumbbells at shoulders, perform deep squat.
	(2) Diamond Push-Ups - 15 reps	Chest, Triceps, Core	Push-up with hands under shoulders, elbows tight.
	(3) Dumbbell Swings - 20 reps	Core, Shoulders, Back	Swing dumbbell between legs then up to shoulder height.
108	**4 Rounds:**		
	(1) Jump Squats - 1 minute	Legs, Glutes, Cardio	Perform squat then jump, holding dumbbells. Land softly.
	(2) Renegade Rows - 12 reps each arm	Back, Shoulders, Core	Row dumbbell from plank position, switch sides.
	(3) Spider-Man Push-Ups - 1 minute	Chest, Core, Shoulders	Perform push-up, bring knee to elbow, switch sides.
109	**For time:**		
	(1) Dumbbell Bench Press - 20 reps	Chest, Triceps, Shoulders	Press dumbbells from chest to straight arms on a bench.
	(2) Walking Lunges - 15 reps each leg	Legs, Glutes, Core	Step forward into lunge holding dumbbells, switch legs.
	(3) Dumbbell Thrusters - 15 reps	Legs, Shoulders, Core	Squat down holding dumbbells at shoulders, explode up and press
110	**6 Rounds:**		
	(1) Tuck Jumps - 45 seconds	Legs, Cardio, Core	Jump high, tuck knees to chest mid-air. Land softly.
	(2) Dumbbell Plank T - 12 reps each side	Core, Shoulders, Back	Rotate into T position from plank with dumbbell, switch sides.
	(3) Push-Ups - 30 seconds	Chest, Triceps, Core	Lower chest to ground, push back up. Keep body straight.
111	**As many rounds as possible in 15 mins of:**		
	(1) Dumbbell Deadlift - 15 reps	Back, Legs, Core	Lower dumbbells to shins with slight knee bend, then lift. Keep back straight.
	(2) Push-Ups - 20 reps	Chest, Triceps, Core	Lower chest to ground, push back up. Keep body straight.
	(3) Dumbbell Step-Ups - 12 reps each leg	Legs, Glutes, Core	Step onto platform holding dumbbells, alternate legs.
112	**5 Rounds:**		
	(1) Jumping Jacks - 1 minute	Cardio, Legs, Shoulders	Jump feet out and clap hands overhead, return quickly. Maintain speed and light
	(2) Dumbbell Thrusters - 12 reps	Legs, Shoulders, Core	Squat down holding dumbbells at shoulders, explode up and press
	(3) Burpees - 1 minute	Full Body, Cardio, Core	Jump, drop into push-up position, perform push-up, jump back up.

Workout No.	Workout (Dumbbell and Body-Weight)	Main Muscle Groups	Instructions
113	**As many rounds as possible in 12 mins of:**		
	(1) Dumbbell Snatch - 10 reps each arm	Shoulders, Back, Core	Lift dumbbell from floor to overhead in one movement, alternate arms.
	(2) Sit-Ups - 20 reps	Abs, Core, Hip Flexors	Lie back, sit up and touch toes. Control descent.
	(3) Dumbbell Lunges - 12 reps each leg	Legs, Glutes, Core	Step forward into lunge holding dumbbells, switch legs.
114	**4 Rounds:**		
	(1) High Knees - 45 seconds	Cardio, Legs, Core	Run in place lifting knees high, maintain pace.
	(2) Dumbbell Shoulder Press - 15 reps	Shoulders, Triceps, Core	Press dumbbells overhead from shoulders, keep core tight.
	(3) V-Ups - 45 seconds	Abs, Core, Hip Flexors	Lie back, lift legs and torso simultaneously, form 'V'.
115	**For time:**		
	(1) Dumbbell Clean and Press - 15 reps	Full Body, Shoulders, Core	Lift dumbbells to shoulders from floor, press overhead.
	(2) Hand-Release Push-Ups - 20 reps	Chest, Triceps, Core	Lower chest to ground, lift hands, push back up.
	(3) Dumbbell Side Lunges - 12 reps each leg	Legs, Glutes, Core	Step sideways into lunge holding dumbbells, switch sides.
116	**5 Rounds:**		
	(1) Burpees - 30 seconds	Full Body, Cardio, Core	Jump, drop into push-up position, perform push-up, jump back up.
	(2) Dumbbell Rows - 15 reps each arm	Back, Biceps, Core	Row dumbbell to hip while bent over, switch sides.
	(3) Mountain Climbers - 30 seconds	Cardio, Core, Shoulders	Run in place in plank position, drive knees to chest.
117	**3 Rounds for time:**		
	(1) Dumbbell Front Squats - 20 reps	Legs, Glutes, Core	Hold dumbbells at shoulders, perform deep squat.
	(2) Diamond Push-Ups - 15 reps	Chest, Triceps, Core	Push-up with hands under shoulders, elbows tight.
	(3) Dumbbell Swings - 20 reps	Core, Shoulders, Back	Swing dumbbell between legs then up to shoulder height.
118	**4 Rounds:**		
	(1) Jump Squats - 1 minute	Legs, Glutes, Cardio	Perform squat then jump, holding dumbbells. Land softly.
	(2) Renegade Rows - 12 reps each arm	Back, Shoulders, Core	Row dumbbell from plank position, switch sides.
	(3) Spider-Man Push-Ups - 1 minute	Chest, Core, Shoulders	Perform push-up, bring knee to elbow, switch sides.
119	**For time:**		
	(1) Dumbbell Bench Press - 20 reps	Chest, Triceps, Shoulders	Press dumbbells from chest to straight arms on a bench.
	(2) Walking Lunges - 15 reps each leg	Legs, Glutes, Core	Step forward into lunge holding dumbbells, switch legs.
	(3) Dumbbell Thrusters - 15 reps	Legs, Shoulders, Core	Squat down holding dumbbells at shoulders, explode up and press
120	**6 Rounds:**		
	(1) Tuck Jumps - 45 seconds	Legs, Cardio, Core	Jump high, tuck knees to chest mid-air. Land softly.
	(2) Dumbbell Plank T - 12 reps each side	Core, Shoulders, Back	Rotate into T position from plank with dumbbell, switch sides.
	(3) Push-Ups - 30 seconds	Chest, Triceps, Core	Lower chest to ground, push back up. Keep body straight.

Workout No.	Workout (Dumbbell and Body-Weight)	Main Muscle Groups	Instructions
121	As many rounds as possible in 15 mins of:		
	(1) Dumbbell Deadlift - 15 reps	Back, Legs, Core	Lower dumbbells to shins with slight knee bend, then lift. Keep back straight.
	(2) Push-Ups - 20 reps	Chest, Triceps, Core	Lower chest to ground, push back up. Keep body straight.
	(3) Dumbbell Step-Ups - 12 reps each leg	Legs, Glutes, Core	Step onto platform holding dumbbells, alternate legs.
122	5 Rounds:		
	(1) Jumping Jacks - 1 minute	Cardio, Legs, Shoulders	Jump feet out and clap hands overhead, return quickly. Maintain speed and light
	(2) Dumbbell Thrusters - 12 reps	Legs, Shoulders, Core	Squat down holding dumbbells at shoulders, explode up and press
	(3) Burpees - 1 minute	Full Body, Cardio, Core	Jump, drop into push-up position, perform push-up, jump back up.
123	As many rounds as possible in 12 mins of:		
	(1) Dumbbell Snatch - 10 reps each arm	Shoulders, Back, Core	Lift dumbbell from floor to overhead in one movement, alternate arms.
	(2) Sit-Ups - 20 reps	Abs, Core, Hip Flexors	Lie back, sit up and touch toes. Control descent.
	(3) Dumbbell Lunges - 12 reps each leg	Legs, Glutes, Core	Step forward into lunge holding dumbbells, switch legs.
124	4 Rounds:		
	(1) High Knees - 45 seconds	Cardio, Legs, Core	Run in place lifting knees high, maintain pace.
	(2) Dumbbell Shoulder Press - 15 reps	Shoulders, Triceps, Core	Press dumbbells overhead from shoulders, keep core tight.
	(3) V-Ups - 45 seconds	Abs, Core, Hip Flexors	Lie back, lift legs and torso simultaneously, form 'V'.
125	For time:		
	(1) Dumbbell Clean and Press - 15 reps	Full Body, Shoulders, Core	Lift dumbbells to shoulders from floor, press overhead.
	(2) Hand-Release Push-Ups - 20 reps	Chest, Triceps, Core	Lower chest to ground, lift hands, push back up.
	(3) Dumbbell Side Lunges - 12 reps each leg	Legs, Glutes, Core	Step sideways into lunge holding dumbbells, switch sides.
126	5 Rounds:		
	(1) Burpees - 30 seconds	Full Body, Cardio, Core	Jump, drop into push-up position, perform push-up, jump back up.
	(2) Dumbbell Rows - 15 reps each arm	Back, Biceps, Core	Row dumbbell to hip while bent over, switch sides.
	(3) Mountain Climbers - 30 seconds	Cardio, Core, Shoulders	Run in place in plank position, drive knees to chest.
127	3 Rounds for time:		
	(1) Dumbbell Front Squats - 20 reps	Legs, Glutes, Core	Hold dumbbells at shoulders, perform deep squat.
	(2) Diamond Push-Ups - 15 reps	Chest, Triceps, Core	Push-up with hands under shoulders, elbows tight.
	(3) Dumbbell Swings - 20 reps	Core, Shoulders, Back	Swing dumbbell between legs then up to shoulder height.
128	4 Rounds:		
	(1) Jump Squats - 1 minute	Legs, Glutes, Cardio	Perform squat then jump, holding dumbbells. Land softly.
	(2) Renegade Rows - 12 reps each arm	Back, Shoulders, Core	Row dumbbell from plank position, switch sides.
	(3) Spider-Man Push-Ups - 1 minute	Chest, Core, Shoulders	Perform push-up, bring knee to elbow, switch sides.

Workout No.	Workout (Dumbbell and Body-Weight)	Main Muscle Groups	Instructions
129	**For time:**		
	(1) Dumbbell Bench Press - 20 reps	Chest, Triceps, Shoulders	Press dumbbells from chest to straight arms on a bench.
	(2) Walking Lunges - 15 reps each leg	Legs, Glutes, Core	Step forward into lunge holding dumbbells, switch legs.
	(3) Dumbbell Thrusters - 15 reps	Legs, Shoulders, Core	Squat down holding dumbbells at shoulders, explode up and press
130	**6 Rounds:**		
	(1) Tuck Jumps - 45 seconds	Legs, Cardio, Core	Jump high, tuck knees to chest mid-air. Land softly.
	(2) Dumbbell Plank T - 12 reps each side	Core, Shoulders, Back	Rotate into T position from plank with dumbbell, switch sides.
	(3) Push-Ups - 30 seconds	Chest, Triceps, Core	Lower chest to ground, push back up. Keep body straight.
131	**As many rounds as possible in 15 mins of:**		
	(1) Dumbbell Deadlift - 15 reps	Back, Legs, Core	Lower dumbbells to shins with slight knee bend, then lift. Keep back straight.
	(2) Push-Ups - 20 reps	Chest, Triceps, Core	Lower chest to ground, push back up. Keep body straight.
	(3) Dumbbell Step-Ups - 12 reps each leg	Legs, Glutes, Core	Step onto platform holding dumbbells, alternate legs.
132	**5 Rounds:**		
	(1) Jumping Jacks - 1 minute	Cardio, Legs, Shoulders	Jump feet out and clap hands overhead, return quickly. Maintain speed and light
	(2) Dumbbell Thrusters - 12 reps	Legs, Shoulders, Core	Squat down holding dumbbells at shoulders, explode up and press
	(3) Burpees - 1 minute	Full Body, Cardio, Core	Jump, drop into push-up position, perform push-up, jump back up.
133	**As many rounds as possible in 12 mins of:**		
	(1) Dumbbell Snatch - 10 reps each arm	Shoulders, Back, Core	Lift dumbbell from floor to overhead in one movement, alternate arms.
	(2) Sit-Ups - 20 reps	Abs, Core, Hip Flexors	Lie back, sit up and touch toes. Control descent.
	(3) Dumbbell Lunges - 12 reps each leg	Legs, Glutes, Core	Step forward into lunge holding dumbbells, switch legs.
134	**4 Rounds:**		
	(1) High Knees - 45 seconds	Cardio, Legs, Core	Run in place lifting knees high, maintain pace.
	(2) Dumbbell Shoulder Press - 15 reps	Shoulders, Triceps, Core	Press dumbbells overhead from shoulders, keep core tight.
	(3) V-Ups - 45 seconds	Abs, Core, Hip Flexors	Lie back, lift legs and torso simultaneously, form 'V'.
135	**For time:**		
	(1) Dumbbell Clean and Press - 15 reps	Full Body, Shoulders, Core	Lift dumbbells to shoulders from floor, press overhead.
	(2) Hand-Release Push-Ups - 20 reps	Chest, Triceps, Core	Lower chest to ground, lift hands, push back up.
	(3) Dumbbell Side Lunges - 12 reps each leg	Legs, Glutes, Core	Step sideways into lunge holding dumbbells, switch sides.
136	**5 Rounds:**		
	(1) Burpees - 30 seconds	Full Body, Cardio, Core	Jump, drop into push-up position, perform push-up, jump back up.
	(2) Dumbbell Rows - 15 reps each arm	Back, Biceps, Core	Row dumbbell to hip while bent over, switch sides.
	(3) Mountain Climbers - 30 seconds	Cardio, Core, Shoulders	Run in place in plank position, drive knees to chest.

Workout No.	Workout (Dumbbell and Body-Weight)	Main Muscle Groups	Instructions
137	**3 Rounds for time:**		
	(1) Dumbbell Front Squats - 20 reps	Legs, Glutes, Core	Hold dumbbells at shoulders, perform deep squat.
	(2) Diamond Push-Ups - 15 reps	Chest, Triceps, Core	Push-up with hands under shoulders, elbows tight.
	(3) Dumbbell Swings - 20 reps	Core, Shoulders, Back	Swing dumbbell between legs then up to shoulder height.
138	**4 Rounds:**		
	(1) Jump Squats - 1 minute	Legs, Glutes, Cardio	Perform squat then jump, holding dumbbells. Land softly.
	(2) Renegade Rows - 12 reps each arm	Back, Shoulders, Core	Row dumbbell from plank position, switch sides.
	(3) Spider-Man Push-Ups - 1 minute	Chest, Core, Shoulders	Perform push-up, bring knee to elbow, switch sides.
139	**For time:**		
	(1) Dumbbell Bench Press - 20 reps	Chest, Triceps, Shoulders	Press dumbbells from chest to straight arms on a bench.
	(2) Walking Lunges - 15 reps each leg	Legs, Glutes, Core	Step forward into lunge holding dumbbells, switch legs.
	(3) Dumbbell Thrusters - 15 reps	Legs, Shoulders, Core	Squat down holding dumbbells at shoulders, explode up and press
140	**6 Rounds:**		
	(1) Tuck Jumps - 45 seconds	Legs, Cardio, Core	Jump high, tuck knees to chest mid-air. Land softly.
	(2) Dumbbell Plank T - 12 reps each side	Core, Shoulders, Back	Rotate into T position from plank with dumbbell, switch sides.
	(3) Push-Ups - 30 seconds	Chest, Triceps, Core	Lower chest to ground, push back up. Keep body straight.
141	**As many rounds as possible in 15 mins of:**		
	(1) Dumbbell Deadlift - 15 reps	Back, Legs, Core	Lower dumbbells to shins with slight knee bend, then lift. Keep back straight.
	(2) Push-Ups - 20 reps	Chest, Triceps, Core	Lower chest to ground, push back up. Keep body straight.
	(3) Dumbbell Step-Ups - 12 reps each leg	Legs, Glutes, Core	Step onto platform holding dumbbells, alternate legs.
142	**5 Rounds:**		
	(1) Jumping Jacks - 1 minute	Cardio, Legs, Shoulders	Jump feet out and clap hands overhead, return quickly. Maintain speed and light
	(2) Dumbbell Thrusters - 12 reps	Legs, Shoulders, Core	Squat down holding dumbbells at shoulders, explode up and press
	(3) Burpees - 1 minute	Full Body, Cardio, Core	Jump, drop into push-up position, perform push-up, jump back up.
143	**As many rounds as possible in 12 mins of:**		
	(1) Dumbbell Snatch - 10 reps each arm	Shoulders, Back, Core	Lift dumbbell from floor to overhead in one movement, alternate arms.
	(2) Sit-Ups - 20 reps	Abs, Core, Hip Flexors	Lie back, sit up and touch toes. Control descent.
	(3) Dumbbell Lunges - 12 reps each leg	Legs, Glutes, Core	Step forward into lunge holding dumbbells, switch legs.
144	**4 Rounds:**		
	(1) High Knees - 45 seconds	Cardio, Legs, Core	Run in place lifting knees high, maintain pace.
	(2) Dumbbell Shoulder Press - 15 reps	Shoulders, Triceps, Core	Press dumbbells overhead from shoulders, keep core tight.
	(3) V-Ups - 45 seconds	Abs, Core, Hip Flexors	Lie back, lift legs and torso simultaneously, form 'V'.

Workout No.	Workout (Dumbbell and Body-Weight)	Main Muscle Groups	Instructions
145	**For time:**		
	(1) Dumbbell Clean and Press - 15 reps	Full Body, Shoulders, Core	Lift dumbbells to shoulders from floor, press overhead.
	(2) Hand-Release Push-Ups - 20 reps	Chest, Triceps, Core	Lower chest to ground, lift hands, push back up.
	(3) Dumbbell Side Lunges - 12 reps each leg	Legs, Glutes, Core	Step sideways into lunge holding dumbbells, switch sides.
146	**5 Rounds:**		
	(1) Burpees - 30 seconds	Full Body, Cardio, Core	Jump, drop into push-up position, perform push-up, jump back up.
	(2) Dumbbell Rows - 15 reps each arm	Back, Biceps, Core	Row dumbbell to hip while bent over, switch sides.
	(3) Mountain Climbers - 30 seconds	Cardio, Core, Shoulders	Run in place in plank position, drive knees to chest.
147	**3 Rounds for time:**		
	(1) Dumbbell Front Squats - 20 reps	Legs, Glutes, Core	Hold dumbbells at shoulders, perform deep squat.
	(2) Diamond Push-Ups - 15 reps	Chest, Triceps, Core	Push-up with hands under shoulders, elbows tight.
	(3) Dumbbell Swings - 20 reps	Core, Shoulders, Back	Swing dumbbell between legs then up to shoulder height.
148	**4 Rounds:**		
	(1) Jump Squats - 1 minute	Legs, Glutes, Cardio	Perform squat then jump, holding dumbbells. Land softly.
	(2) Renegade Rows - 12 reps each arm	Back, Shoulders, Core	Row dumbbell from plank position, switch sides.
	(3) Spider-Man Push-Ups - 1 minute	Chest, Core, Shoulders	Perform push-up, bring knee to elbow, switch sides.
149	**For time:**		
	(1) Dumbbell Bench Press - 20 reps	Chest, Triceps, Shoulders	Press dumbbells from chest to straight arms on a bench.
	(2) Walking Lunges - 15 reps each leg	Legs, Glutes, Core	Step forward into lunge holding dumbbells, switch legs.
	(3) Dumbbell Thrusters - 15 reps	Legs, Shoulders, Core	Squat down holding dumbbells at shoulders, explode up and press
150	**6 Rounds:**		
	(1) Tuck Jumps - 45 seconds	Legs, Cardio, Core	Jump high, tuck knees to chest mid-air. Land softly.
	(2) Dumbbell Plank T - 12 reps each side	Core, Shoulders, Back	Rotate into T position from plank with dumbbell, switch sides.
	(3) Push-Ups - 30 seconds	Chest, Triceps, Core	Lower chest to ground, push back up. Keep body straight.

Part III

150 Kettlebell Only Workouts

Workout No.	Workout (Kettlebell ONLY workouts)	Main Muscle Groups	Instructions
1	**As many rounds as possible in 10 mins of:**		
	(1) 10 Goblet Squats	Quads, Glutes, Core	Hold kettlebell at chest, squat, keep back straight.
	(2) 10 Kettlebell Swings	Hamstrings, Glutes, Shoulders	Swing kettlebell to chest height, hinge at hips.
	(3) 10 Push Press	Shoulders, Triceps, Core	Push kettlebell overhead, lock out arms.
2	**Every minute on the minute for 20 mins:**		
	(1) 15 Kettlebell Snatches (Alternating)	Shoulders, Glutes, Hamstrings	Lift kettlebell overhead in one motion, switch hands.
	(2) 20 Russian Twists	Obliques, Core, Shoulders	Twist torso, touch kettlebell to ground each side.
3	**3 Rounds for time:**		
	(1) 15 Kettlebell Cleans	Shoulders, Biceps, Core	Lift kettlebell to shoulder, flip grip at top.
	(2) 20 Kettlebell Deadlifts	Hamstrings, Glutes, Back	Lift kettlebell from ground, keep back straight.
	(3) 15 Pushups on Kettlebell	Chest, Triceps, Shoulders	Perform pushup with hands on kettlebell.
4	**45 secs work / 15 secs rest per exercise for 4 rounds:**		
	(1) Kettlebell Thrusters	Quads, Shoulders, Triceps	Squat to overhead press, one fluid motion.
	(2) Bent Over Rows	Back, Biceps, Core	Row kettlebell to hip, switch sides.
	(3) Kettlebell Jump Swings	Hamstrings, Glutes, Core	Swing kettlebell with a jump at top of motion.
5	**5 Rounds for time:**		
	(1) 10 Turkish GetUps	Shoulders, Core, Legs	Stand from floor, kettlebell overhead, controlled motion.
	(2) 15 Goblet Squats	Quads, Glutes, Core	Hold kettlebell at chest, squat, keep back straight.
	(3) 10 Burpees over Kettlebell	Full Body, Cardio	Perform burpee, jump over kettlebell.

Workout No.	Workout (Kettlebell ONLY workouts)	Main Muscle Groups	Instructions
6	**As many rounds as possible in 10 mins:**		
	(1) 20 Kettlebell Swings	Hamstrings, Glutes, Shoulders	Swing kettlebell to chest height, hinge at hips.
	(2) 15 Kettlebell Lunges (Alternating)	Quads, Glutes, Core	Step forward into lunge, hold kettlebell for balance.
	(3) 10 Renegade Rows	Back, Biceps, Core	Row kettlebells alternately in plank position.
7	**21-15-9 Reps for time:**		
	(1) Kettlebell Cleans	Shoulders, Biceps, Core	Lift kettlebell to shoulder, flip grip at top.
	(2) Kettlebell Swings	Hamstrings, Glutes, Shoulders	Swing kettlebell to chest height, hinge at hips.
	(3) Kettlebell Push Press	Shoulders, Triceps, Core	Push kettlebell overhead, lock out arms.
8	**Every minute on the minute for 25 mins:**		
	(1) 20 Kettlebell Deadlifts	Hamstrings, Glutes, Back	Lift kettlebell from ground, keep back straight.
	(2) 20 Alternating Kettlebell Lunges	Quads, Glutes, Core	Step forward into lunge, hold kettlebell for balance.
	(3) 10 Kettlebell Thrusters	Quads, Shoulders, Triceps	Squat to overhead press, one fluid motion.
9	**As many rounds as possible in 12 mins:**		
	(1) 10 Goblet Squats	Quads, Glutes, Core	Hold kettlebell at chest, squat, keep back straight.
	(2) 15 Russian Twists	Obliques, Core, Shoulders	Twist torso, touch kettlebell to ground each side.
	(3) 10 Kettlebell Snatches	Shoulders, Glutes, Hamstrings	Lift kettlebell overhead in one motion, switch hands.
10	**4 Rounds for time:**		
	(1) 10 Kettlebell Thrusters	Quads, Shoulders, Triceps	Squat to overhead press, one fluid motion.
	(2) 15 Bent Over Rows	Back, Biceps, Core	Row kettlebell to hip, switch sides.
	(3) 20 Russian Twists	Obliques, Core, Shoulders	Twist torso, touch kettlebell to ground each side.

Workout No.	Workout (Kettlebell ONLY workouts)	Main Muscle Groups	Instructions
11	**As many rounds as possible in 12 min:**		
	(1) 10 Goblet Squats	Quads, Glutes, Core	Hold kettlebell at chest, squat, keep back straight.
	(2) 10 Kettlebell Swings	Hamstrings, Glutes, Shoulders	Swing kettlebell to chest height, hinge at hips.
	(3) 10 Push Press	Shoulders, Triceps, Core	Push kettlebell overhead, lock out arms.
12	**Every minute on the minute for 20 mins:**		
	(1) 15 Kettlebell Snatches (Alternating)	Shoulders, Glutes, Hamstrings	Lift kettlebell overhead in one motion, switch hands.
	(2) 20 Russian Twists	Obliques, Core, Shoulders	Twist torso, touch kettlebell to ground each side.
13	**3 Rounds for time:**		
	(1) 15 Kettlebell Cleans	Shoulders, Biceps, Core	Lift kettlebell to shoulder, flip grip at top.
	(2) 20 Kettlebell Deadlifts	Hamstrings, Glutes, Back	Lift kettlebell from ground, keep back straight.
	(3) 15 Pushups on Kettlebell	Chest, Triceps, Shoulders	Perform pushup with hands on kettlebell.
14	**45 secs work / 15 secs rest per exercise for 4 rounds:**		
	(1) Kettlebell Thrusters	Quads, Shoulders, Triceps	Squat to overhead press, one fluid motion.
	(2) Bent Over Rows	Back, Biceps, Core	Row kettlebell to hip, switch sides.
	(3) Kettlebell Jump Swings	Hamstrings, Glutes, Core	Swing kettlebell with a jump at top of motion.
15	**5 Rounds for time:**		
	(1) 10 Turkish GetUps	Shoulders, Core, Legs	Stand from floor, kettlebell overhead, controlled motion.
	(2) 15 Goblet Squats	Quads, Glutes, Core	Hold kettlebell at chest, squat, keep back straight.
	(3) 10 Burpees over Kettlebell	Full Body, Cardio	Perform burpee, jump over kettlebell.

Workout No.	Workout (Kettlebell ONLY workouts)	Main Muscle Groups	Instructions
16	**As many rounds as possible in 10 mins:**		
	(1) 20 Kettlebell Swings	Hamstrings, Glutes, Shoulders	Swing kettlebell to chest height, hinge at hips.
	(2) 15 Kettlebell Lunges (Alternating)	Quads, Glutes, Core	Step forward into lunge, hold kettlebell for balance.
	(3) 10 Renegade Rows	Back, Biceps, Core	Row kettlebells alternately in plank position.
17	**21-15-9 Reps for time:**		
	(1) Kettlebell Cleans	Shoulders, Biceps, Core	Lift kettlebell to shoulder, flip grip at top.
	(2) Kettlebell Swings	Hamstrings, Glutes, Shoulders	Swing kettlebell to chest height, hinge at hips.
	(3) Kettlebell Push Press	Shoulders, Triceps, Core	Push kettlebell overhead, lock out arms.
18	**Every minute on the minute for 25 mins:**		
	(1) 20 Kettlebell Deadlifts	Hamstrings, Glutes, Back	Lift kettlebell from ground, keep back straight.
	(2) 20 Alternating Kettlebell Lunges	Quads, Glutes, Core	Step forward into lunge, hold kettlebell for balance.
	(3) 10 Kettlebell Thrusters	Quads, Shoulders, Triceps	Squat to overhead press, one fluid motion.
19	**As many rounds as possible in 12 mins:**		
	(1) 10 Goblet Squats	Quads, Glutes, Core	Hold kettlebell at chest, squat, keep back straight.
	(2) 15 Russian Twists	Obliques, Core, Shoulders	Twist torso, touch kettlebell to ground each side.
	(3) 10 Kettlebell Snatches	Shoulders, Glutes, Hamstrings	Lift kettlebell overhead in one motion, switch hands.
20	**4 Rounds for time:**		
	(1) 10 Kettlebell Thrusters	Quads, Shoulders, Triceps	Squat to overhead press, one fluid motion.
	(2) 15 Bent Over Rows	Back, Biceps, Core	Row kettlebell to hip, switch sides.
	(3) 20 Russian Twists	Obliques, Core, Shoulders	Twist torso, touch kettlebell to ground each side.

Workout No.	Workout (Kettlebell ONLY workouts)	Main Muscle Groups	Instructions
21	**As many rounds as possible in 15 min:**		
	(1) 10 Goblet Squats	Quads, Glutes, Core	Hold kettlebell at chest, squat, keep back straight.
	(2) 10 Kettlebell Swings	Hamstrings, Glutes, Shoulders	Swing kettlebell to chest height, hinge at hips.
	(3) 10 Push Press	Shoulders, Triceps, Core	Push kettlebell overhead, lock out arms.
22	**Every minute on the minute for 20 mins:**		
	(1) 12 Kettlebell Snatches (Alternating)	Shoulders, Glutes, Hamstrings	Lift kettlebell overhead in one motion, switch hands.
	(2) 16 Russian Twists	Obliques, Core, Shoulders	Twist torso, touch kettlebell to ground each side.
23	**4 Rounds for time:**		
	(1) 20 Kettlebell Cleans	Shoulders, Biceps, Core	Lift kettlebell to shoulder, flip grip at top.
	(2) 15 Kettlebell Deadlifts	Hamstrings, Glutes, Back	Lift kettlebell from ground, keep back straight.
	(3) 20 Pushups on Kettlebell	Chest, Triceps, Shoulders	Perform pushup with hands on kettlebell.
24	**45 secs work / 15 secs rest per exercise for 5 rounds:**		
	(1) Kettlebell Thrusters	Quads, Shoulders, Triceps	Squat to overhead press, one fluid motion.
	(2) Bent Over Rows	Back, Biceps, Core	Row kettlebell to hip, switch sides.
	(3) Kettlebell Jump Swings	Hamstrings, Glutes, Core	Swing kettlebell with a jump at top of motion.
25	**5 Rounds for time:**		
	(1) 10 Turkish GetUps	Shoulders, Core, Legs	Stand from floor, kettlebell overhead, controlled motion.
	(2) 20 Goblet Squats	Quads, Glutes, Core	Hold kettlebell at chest, squat, keep back straight.
	(3) 15 Burpees over Kettlebell	Full Body, Cardio	Perform burpee, jump over kettlebell.

Workout No.	Workout (Kettlebell ONLY workouts)	Main Muscle Groups	Instructions
26	**As many rounds as possible in 12 mins:**		
	(1) 15 Kettlebell Swings	Hamstrings, Glutes, Shoulders	Swing kettlebell to chest height, hinge at hips.
	(2) 12 Kettlebell Lunges (Alternating)	Quads, Glutes, Core	Step forward into lunge, hold kettlebell for balance.
	(3) 10 Renegade Rows	Back, Biceps, Core	Row kettlebells alternately in plank position.
27	**21-15-9 Reps for time:**		
	(1) Kettlebell Cleans	Shoulders, Biceps, Core	Lift kettlebell to shoulder, flip grip at top.
	(2) Kettlebell Swings	Hamstrings, Glutes, Shoulders	Swing kettlebell to chest height, hinge at hips.
	(3) Kettlebell Push Press	Shoulders, Triceps, Core	Push kettlebell overhead, lock out arms.
28	**Every minute on the minute for 25 mins:**		
	(1) 15 Kettlebell Deadlifts	Hamstrings, Glutes, Back	Lift kettlebell from ground, keep back straight.
	(2) 12 Alternating Kettlebell Lunges	Quads, Glutes, Core	Step forward into lunge, hold kettlebell for balance.
	(3) 10 Kettlebell Thrusters	Quads, Shoulders, Triceps	Squat to overhead press, one fluid motion.
29	**As many rounds as possible in 12 mins:**		
	(1) 10 Goblet Squats	Quads, Glutes, Core	Hold kettlebell at chest, squat, keep back straight.
	(2) 20 Russian Twists	Obliques, Core, Shoulders	Twist torso, touch kettlebell to ground each side.
	(3) 15 Kettlebell Snatches	Shoulders, Glutes, Hamstrings	Lift kettlebell overhead in one motion, switch hands.
30	**5 Rounds for time:**		
	(1) 12 Kettlebell Thrusters	Quads, Shoulders, Triceps	Squat to overhead press, one fluid motion.
	(2) 15 Bent Over Rows	Back, Biceps, Core	Row kettlebell to hip, switch sides.
	(3) 20 Russian Twists	Obliques, Core, Shoulders	Twist torso, touch kettlebell to ground each side.

Workout No.	Workout (Kettlebell ONLY workouts)	Main Muscle Groups	Instructions
31	**As many rounds as possible in 12 min:**		
	(1) 12 Goblet Squats	Quads, Glutes, Core	Hold kettlebell at chest, squat, keep back straight.
	(2) 15 Kettlebell Swings	Hamstrings, Glutes, Shoulders	Swing kettlebell to chest height, hinge at hips.
	(3) 10 Push Press	Shoulders, Triceps, Core	Push kettlebell overhead, lock out arms.
32	**Every minute on the minute for 20 mins:**		
	(1) 12 Kettlebell Snatches (Alternating)	Shoulders, Glutes, Hamstrings	Lift kettlebell overhead in one motion, switch hands.
	(2) 16 Russian Twists	Obliques, Core, Shoulders	Twist torso, touch kettlebell to ground each side.
33	**3 Rounds for time:**		
	(1) 15 Kettlebell Cleans	Shoulders, Biceps, Core	Lift kettlebell to shoulder, flip grip at top.
	(2) 20 Kettlebell Deadlifts	Hamstrings, Glutes, Back	Lift kettlebell from ground, keep back straight.
	(3) 15 Pushups on Kettlebell	Chest, Triceps, Shoulders	Perform pushup with hands on kettlebell.
34	**45 secs work / 15 secs rest per exercise for 4 rounds:**		
	(1) Kettlebell Thrusters	Quads, Shoulders, Triceps	Squat to overhead press, one fluid motion.
	(2) Bent Over Rows	Back, Biceps, Core	Row kettlebell to hip, switch sides.
	(3) Kettlebell Jump Swings	Hamstrings, Glutes, Core	Swing kettlebell with a jump at top of motion.
35	**5 Rounds for time:**		
	(1) 10 Turkish GetUps	Shoulders, Core, Legs	Stand from floor, kettlebell overhead, controlled motion.
	(2) 15 Goblet Squats	Quads, Glutes, Core	Hold kettlebell at chest, squat, keep back straight.
	(3) 10 Burpees over Kettlebell	Full Body, Cardio	Perform burpee, jump over kettlebell.

Workout No.	Workout (Kettlebell ONLY workouts)	Main Muscle Groups	Instructions
36	**As many rounds as possible in 10 mins:**		
	(1) 20 Kettlebell Swings	Hamstrings, Glutes, Shoulders	Swing kettlebell to chest height, hinge at hips.
	(2) 15 Kettlebell Lunges (Alternating)	Quads, Glutes, Core	Step forward into lunge, hold kettlebell for balance.
	(3) 10 Renegade Rows	Back, Biceps, Core	Row kettlebells alternately in plank position.
37	**21-15-9 Reps for time:**		
	(1) Kettlebell Cleans	Shoulders, Biceps, Core	Lift kettlebell to shoulder, flip grip at top.
	(2) Kettlebell Swings	Hamstrings, Glutes, Shoulders	Swing kettlebell to chest height, hinge at hips.
	(3) Kettlebell Push Press	Shoulders, Triceps, Core	Push kettlebell overhead, lock out arms.
38	**Every minute on the minute for 25 mins:**		
	(1) 20 Kettlebell Deadlifts	Hamstrings, Glutes, Back	Lift kettlebell from ground, keep back straight.
	(2) 20 Alternating Kettlebell Lunges	Quads, Glutes, Core	Step forward into lunge, hold kettlebell for balance.
	(3) 10 Kettlebell Thrusters	Quads, Shoulders, Triceps	Squat to overhead press, one fluid motion.
39	**As many rounds as possible in 12 mins:**		
	(1) 10 Goblet Squats	Quads, Glutes, Core	Hold kettlebell at chest, squat, keep back straight.
	(2) 15 Russian Twists	Obliques, Core, Shoulders	Twist torso, touch kettlebell to ground each side.
	(3) 10 Kettlebell Snatches	Shoulders, Glutes, Hamstrings	Lift kettlebell overhead in one motion, switch hands.
40	**4 Rounds for time:**		
	(1) 10 Kettlebell Thrusters	Quads, Shoulders, Triceps	Squat to overhead press, one fluid motion.
	(2) 15 Bent Over Rows	Back, Biceps, Core	Row kettlebell to hip, switch sides.
	(3) 20 Russian Twists	Obliques, Core, Shoulders	Twist torso, touch kettlebell to ground each side.

Workout No.	Workout (Kettlebell ONLY workouts)	Main Muscle Groups	Instructions
41	**As many rounds as possible in 12 min:**		
	(1) 15 Goblet Squats	Quads, Glutes, Core	Hold kettlebell at chest, squat, keep back straight.
	(2) 12 Kettlebell Swings	Hamstrings, Glutes, Shoulders	Swing kettlebell to chest height, hinge at hips.
	(3) 10 Push Press	Shoulders, Triceps, Core	Push kettlebell overhead, lock out arms.
42	**Every minute on the minute for 20 mins:**		
	(1) 12 Kettlebell Snatches (Alternating)	Shoulders, Glutes, Hamstrings	Lift kettlebell overhead in one motion, switch hands.
	(2) 16 Russian Twists	Obliques, Core, Shoulders	Twist torso, touch kettlebell to ground each side.
43	**3 Rounds for time:**		
	(1) 15 Kettlebell Cleans	Shoulders, Biceps, Core	Lift kettlebell to shoulder, flip grip at top.
	(2) 20 Kettlebell Deadlifts	Hamstrings, Glutes, Back	Lift kettlebell from ground, keep back straight.
	(3) 15 Pushups on Kettlebell	Chest, Triceps, Shoulders	Perform pushup with hands on kettlebell.
44	**45 secs work / 15 secs rest per exercise for 4 rounds:**		
	(1) Kettlebell Thrusters	Quads, Shoulders, Triceps	Squat to overhead press, one fluid motion.
	(2) Bent Over Rows	Back, Biceps, Core	Row kettlebell to hip, switch sides.
	(3) Kettlebell Jump Swings	Hamstrings, Glutes, Core	Swing kettlebell with a jump at top of motion.
45	**5 Rounds for time:**		
	(1) 10 Turkish GetUps	Shoulders, Core, Legs	Stand from floor, kettlebell overhead, controlled motion.
	(2) 15 Goblet Squats	Quads, Glutes, Core	Hold kettlebell at chest, squat, keep back straight.
	(3) 10 Burpees over Kettlebell	Full Body, Cardio	Perform burpee, jump over kettlebell.

Workout No.	Workout (Kettlebell ONLY workouts)		Main Muscle Groups	Instructions
46	As many rounds as possible in 10 mins:			
	(1)	20 Kettlebell Swings	Hamstrings, Glutes, Shoulders	Swing kettlebell to chest height, hinge at hips.
	(2)	15 Kettlebell Lunges (Alternating)	Quads, Glutes, Core	Step forward into lunge, hold kettlebell for balance.
	(3)	10 Renegade Rows	Back, Biceps, Core	Row kettlebells alternately in plank position.
47	21-15-9 Reps for time:			
	(1)	Kettlebell Cleans	Shoulders, Biceps, Core	Lift kettlebell to shoulder, flip grip at top.
	(2)	Kettlebell Swings	Hamstrings, Glutes, Shoulders	Swing kettlebell to chest height, hinge at hips.
	(3)	Kettlebell Push Press	Shoulders, Triceps, Core	Push kettlebell overhead, lock out arms.
48	Every minute on the minute for 25 mins:			
	(1)	20 Kettlebell Deadlifts	Hamstrings, Glutes, Back	Lift kettlebell from ground, keep back straight.
	(2)	20 Alternating Kettlebell Lunges	Quads, Glutes, Core	Step forward into lunge, hold kettlebell for balance.
	(3)	10 Kettlebell Thrusters	Quads, Shoulders, Triceps	Squat to overhead press, one fluid motion.
49	As many rounds as possible in 12 mins:			
	(1)	10 Goblet Squats	Quads, Glutes, Core	Hold kettlebell at chest, squat, keep back straight.
	(2)	15 Russian Twists	Obliques, Core, Shoulders	Twist torso, touch kettlebell to ground each side.
	(3)	10 Kettlebell Snatches	Shoulders, Glutes, Hamstrings	Lift kettlebell overhead in one motion, switch hands.
50	4 Rounds for time:			
	(1)	10 Kettlebell Thrusters	Quads, Shoulders, Triceps	Squat to overhead press, one fluid motion.
	(2)	15 Bent Over Rows	Back, Biceps, Core	Row kettlebell to hip, switch sides.
	(3)	20 Russian Twists	Obliques, Core, Shoulders	Twist torso, touch kettlebell to ground each side.

Workout No.	Workout (Kettlebell ONLY workouts)		Main Muscle Groups	Instructions
51	As many rounds as possible in 15 min:			
	(1)	15 Goblet Squats	Quads, Glutes, Core	Hold kettlebell at chest, squat, keep back straight.
	(2)	12 Kettlebell Swings	Hamstrings, Glutes, Shoulders	Swing kettlebell to chest height, hinge at hips.
	(3)	10 Push Press	Shoulders, Triceps, Core	Push kettlebell overhead, lock out arms.
52	Every minute on the minute for 20 mins:			
	(1)	12 Kettlebell Snatches (Alternating)	Shoulders, Glutes, Hamstrings	Lift kettlebell overhead in one motion, switch hands.
	(2)	16 Russian Twists	Obliques, Core, Shoulders	Twist torso, touch kettlebell to ground each side.
53	3 Rounds for time:			
	(1)	15 Kettlebell Cleans	Shoulders, Biceps, Core	Lift kettlebell to shoulder, flip grip at top.
	(2)	20 Kettlebell Deadlifts	Hamstrings, Glutes, Back	Lift kettlebell from ground, keep back straight.
	(3)	15 Pushups on Kettlebell	Chest, Triceps, Shoulders	Perform pushup with hands on kettlebell.
54	45 secs work / 15 secs rest per exercise for 4 rounds:			
	(1)	Kettlebell Thrusters	Quads, Shoulders, Triceps	Squat to overhead press, one fluid motion.
	(2)	Bent Over Rows	Back, Biceps, Core	Row kettlebell to hip, switch sides.
	(3)	Kettlebell Jump Swings	Hamstrings, Glutes, Core	Swing kettlebell with a jump at top of motion.
55	5 Rounds for time:			
	(1)	10 Turkish GetUps	Shoulders, Core, Legs	Stand from floor, kettlebell overhead, controlled motion.
	(2)	15 Goblet Squats	Quads, Glutes, Core	Hold kettlebell at chest, squat, keep back straight.
	(3)	10 Burpees over Kettlebell	Full Body, Cardio	Perform burpee, jump over kettlebell.

Workout No.	Workout (Kettlebell ONLY workouts)		Main Muscle Groups	Instructions
56	As many rounds as possible in 10 mins:			
	(1)	20 Kettlebell Swings	Hamstrings, Glutes, Shoulders	Swing kettlebell to chest height, hinge at hips.
	(2)	15 Kettlebell Lunges (Alternating)	Quads, Glutes, Core	Step forward into lunge, hold kettlebell for balance.
	(3)	10 Renegade Rows	Back, Biceps, Core	Row kettlebells alternately in plank position.
57	21-15-9 Reps for time:			
	(1)	Kettlebell Cleans	Shoulders, Biceps, Core	Lift kettlebell to shoulder, flip grip at top.
	(2)	Kettlebell Swings	Hamstrings, Glutes, Shoulders	Swing kettlebell to chest height, hinge at hips.
	(3)	Kettlebell Push Press	Shoulders, Triceps, Core	Push kettlebell overhead, lock out arms.
58	Every minute on the minute for 25 mins:			
	(1)	20 Kettlebell Deadlifts	Hamstrings, Glutes, Back	Lift kettlebell from ground, keep back straight.
	(2)	20 Alternating Kettlebell Lunges	Quads, Glutes, Core	Step forward into lunge, hold kettlebell for balance.
	(3)	10 Kettlebell Thrusters	Quads, Shoulders, Triceps	Squat to overhead press, one fluid motion.
59	As many rounds as possible in 12 mins:			
	(1)	10 Goblet Squats	Quads, Glutes, Core	Hold kettlebell at chest, squat, keep back straight.
	(2)	15 Russian Twists	Obliques, Core, Shoulders	Twist torso, touch kettlebell to ground each side.
	(3)	10 Kettlebell Snatches	Shoulders, Glutes, Hamstrings	Lift kettlebell overhead in one motion, switch hands.
60	4 Rounds for time:			
	(1)	10 Kettlebell Thrusters	Quads, Shoulders, Triceps	Squat to overhead press, one fluid motion.
	(2)	15 Bent Over Rows	Back, Biceps, Core	Row kettlebell to hip, switch sides.
	(3)	20 Russian Twists	Obliques, Core, Shoulders	Twist torso, touch kettlebell to ground each side.

Workout No.	Workout (Kettlebell ONLY workouts)	Main Muscle Groups	Instructions
61	**As many rounds as possible in 15 min:**		
	(1) 15 Goblet Squats	Quads, Glutes, Core	Hold kettlebell at chest, squat, keep back straight.
	(2) 12 Kettlebell Swings	Hamstrings, Glutes, Shoulders	Swing kettlebell to chest height, hinge at hips.
	(3) 10 Push Press	Shoulders, Triceps, Core	Push kettlebell overhead, lock out arms.
62	**Every minute on the minute for 20 mins:**		
	(1) 12 Kettlebell Snatches (Alternating)	Shoulders, Glutes, Hamstrings	Lift kettlebell overhead in one motion, switch hands.
	(2) 16 Russian Twists	Obliques, Core, Shoulders	Twist torso, touch kettlebell to ground each side.
63	**3 Rounds for time:**		
	(1) 15 Kettlebell Cleans	Shoulders, Biceps, Core	Lift kettlebell to shoulder, flip grip at top.
	(2) 20 Kettlebell Deadlifts	Hamstrings, Glutes, Back	Lift kettlebell from ground, keep back straight.
	(3) 15 Pushups on Kettlebell	Chest, Triceps, Shoulders	Perform pushup with hands on kettlebell.
64	**45 secs work / 15 secs rest per exercise for 4 rounds:**		
	(1) Kettlebell Thrusters	Quads, Shoulders, Triceps	Squat to overhead press, one fluid motion.
	(2) Bent Over Rows	Back, Biceps, Core	Row kettlebell to hip, switch sides.
	(3) Kettlebell Jump Swings	Hamstrings, Glutes, Core	Swing kettlebell with a jump at top of motion.
65	**5 Rounds for time:**		
	(1) 10 Turkish GetUps	Shoulders, Core, Legs	Stand from floor, kettlebell overhead, controlled motion.
	(2) 15 Goblet Squats	Quads, Glutes, Core	Hold kettlebell at chest, squat, keep back straight.
	(3) 10 Burpees over Kettlebell	Full Body, Cardio	Perform burpee, jump over kettlebell.

Workout No.	Workout (Kettlebell ONLY workouts)	Main Muscle Groups	Instructions
66	**As many rounds as possible in 10 mins:**		
	(1) 20 Kettlebell Swings	Hamstrings, Glutes, Shoulders	Swing kettlebell to chest height, hinge at hips.
	(2) 15 Kettlebell Lunges (Alternating)	Quads, Glutes, Core	Step forward into lunge, hold kettlebell for balance.
	(3) 10 Renegade Rows	Back, Biceps, Core	Row kettlebells alternately in plank position.
67	**21-15-9 Reps for time:**		
	(1) Kettlebell Cleans	Shoulders, Biceps, Core	Lift kettlebell to shoulder, flip grip at top.
	(2) Kettlebell Swings	Hamstrings, Glutes, Shoulders	Swing kettlebell to chest height, hinge at hips.
	(3) Kettlebell Push Press	Shoulders, Triceps, Core	Push kettlebell overhead, lock out arms.
68	**Every minute on the minute for 25 mins:**		
	(1) 20 Kettlebell Deadlifts	Hamstrings, Glutes, Back	Lift kettlebell from ground, keep back straight.
	(2) 20 Alternating Kettlebell Lunges	Quads, Glutes, Core	Step forward into lunge, hold kettlebell for balance.
	(3) 10 Kettlebell Thrusters	Quads, Shoulders, Triceps	Squat to overhead press, one fluid motion.
69	**As many rounds as possible in 12 mins:**		
	(1) 10 Goblet Squats	Quads, Glutes, Core	Hold kettlebell at chest, squat, keep back straight.
	(2) 15 Russian Twists	Obliques, Core, Shoulders	Twist torso, touch kettlebell to ground each side.
	(3) 10 Kettlebell Snatches	Shoulders, Glutes, Hamstrings	Lift kettlebell overhead in one motion, switch hands.
70	**4 Rounds for time:**		
	(1) 10 Kettlebell Thrusters	Quads, Shoulders, Triceps	Squat to overhead press, one fluid motion.
	(2) 15 Bent Over Rows	Back, Biceps, Core	Row kettlebell to hip, switch sides.
	(3) 20 Russian Twists	Obliques, Core, Shoulders	Twist torso, touch kettlebell to ground each side.

Workout No.	Workout (Kettlebell ONLY workouts)	Main Muscle Groups	Instructions
71	**As many rounds as possible in 15 min:**		
	(1) 15 Goblet Squats	Quads, Glutes, Core	Hold kettlebell at chest, squat, keep back straight.
	(2) 12 Kettlebell Swings	Hamstrings, Glutes, Shoulders	Swing kettlebell to chest height, hinge at hips.
	(3) 10 Push Press	Shoulders, Triceps, Core	Push kettlebell overhead, lock out arms.
72	**Every minute on the minute for 20 mins:**		
	(1) 12 Kettlebell Snatches (Alternating)	Shoulders, Glutes, Hamstrings	Lift kettlebell overhead in one motion, switch hands.
	(2) 16 Russian Twists	Obliques, Core, Shoulders	Twist torso, touch kettlebell to ground each side.
73	**3 Rounds for time:**		
	(1) 15 Kettlebell Cleans	Shoulders, Biceps, Core	Lift kettlebell to shoulder, flip grip at top.
	(2) 20 Kettlebell Deadlifts	Hamstrings, Glutes, Back	Lift kettlebell from ground, keep back straight.
	(3) 15 Pushups on Kettlebell	Chest, Triceps, Shoulders	Perform pushup with hands on kettlebell.
74	**45 secs work / 15 secs rest per exercise for 4 rounds:**		
	(1) Kettlebell Thrusters	Quads, Shoulders, Triceps	Squat to overhead press, one fluid motion.
	(2) Bent Over Rows	Back, Biceps, Core	Row kettlebell to hip, switch sides.
	(3) Kettlebell Jump Swings	Hamstrings, Glutes, Core	Swing kettlebell with a jump at top of motion.
75	**5 Rounds for time:**		
	(1) 10 Turkish GetUps	Shoulders, Core, Legs	Stand from floor, kettlebell overhead, controlled motion.
	(2) 15 Goblet Squats	Quads, Glutes, Core	Hold kettlebell at chest, squat, keep back straight.
	(3) 10 Burpees over Kettlebell	Full Body, Cardio	Perform burpee, jump over kettlebell.

Workout No.	Workout (Kettlebell ONLY workouts)	Main Muscle Groups	Instructions
76	**As many rounds as possible in 10 mins:**		
	(1) 20 Kettlebell Swings	Hamstrings, Glutes, Shoulders	Swing kettlebell to chest height, hinge at hips.
	(2) 15 Kettlebell Lunges (Alternating)	Quads, Glutes, Core	Step forward into lunge, hold kettlebell for balance.
	(3) 10 Renegade Rows	Back, Biceps, Core	Row kettlebells alternately in plank position.
77	**21-15-9 Reps for time:**		
	(1) Kettlebell Cleans	Shoulders, Biceps, Core	Lift kettlebell to shoulder, flip grip at top.
	(2) Kettlebell Swings	Hamstrings, Glutes, Shoulders	Swing kettlebell to chest height, hinge at hips.
	(3) Kettlebell Push Press	Shoulders, Triceps, Core	Push kettlebell overhead, lock out arms.
78	**Every minute on the minute for 25 mins:**		
	(1) 20 Kettlebell Deadlifts	Hamstrings, Glutes, Back	Lift kettlebell from ground, keep back straight.
	(2) 20 Alternating Kettlebell Lunges	Quads, Glutes, Core	Step forward into lunge, hold kettlebell for balance.
	(3) 10 Kettlebell Thrusters	Quads, Shoulders, Triceps	Squat to overhead press, one fluid motion.
79	**As many rounds as possible in 12 mins:**		
	(1) 10 Goblet Squats	Quads, Glutes, Core	Hold kettlebell at chest, squat, keep back straight.
	(2) 15 Russian Twists	Obliques, Core, Shoulders	Twist torso, touch kettlebell to ground each side.
	(3) 10 Kettlebell Snatches	Shoulders, Glutes, Hamstrings	Lift kettlebell overhead in one motion, switch hands.
80	**4 Rounds for time:**		
	(1) 10 Kettlebell Thrusters	Quads, Shoulders, Triceps	Squat to overhead press, one fluid motion.
	(2) 15 Bent Over Rows	Back, Biceps, Core	Row kettlebell to hip, switch sides.
	(3) 20 Russian Twists	Obliques, Core, Shoulders	Twist torso, touch kettlebell to ground each side.

Workout No.	Workout (Kettlebell ONLY workouts)	Main Muscle Groups	Instructions
81	**As many rounds as possible in 15 min:**		
	(1) 15 Goblet Squats	Quads, Glutes, Core	Hold kettlebell at chest, squat, keep back straight.
	(2) 12 Kettlebell Swings	Hamstrings, Glutes, Shoulders	Swing kettlebell to chest height, hinge at hips.
	(3) 10 Push Press	Shoulders, Triceps, Core	Push kettlebell overhead, lock out arms.
82	**Every minute on the minute for 20 mins:**		
	(1) 12 Kettlebell Snatches (Alternating)	Shoulders, Glutes, Hamstrings	Lift kettlebell overhead in one motion, switch hands.
	(2) 16 Russian Twists	Obliques, Core, Shoulders	Twist torso, touch kettlebell to ground each side.
83	**3 Rounds for time:**		
	(1) 15 Kettlebell Cleans	Shoulders, Biceps, Core	Lift kettlebell to shoulder, flip grip at top.
	(2) 20 Kettlebell Deadlifts	Hamstrings, Glutes, Back	Lift kettlebell from ground, keep back straight.
	(3) 15 Pushups on Kettlebell	Chest, Triceps, Shoulders	Perform pushup with hands on kettlebell.
84	**45 secs work / 15 secs rest per exercise for 4 rounds:**		
	(1) Kettlebell Thrusters	Quads, Shoulders, Triceps	Squat to overhead press, one fluid motion.
	(2) Bent Over Rows	Back, Biceps, Core	Row kettlebell to hip, switch sides.
	(3) Kettlebell Jump Swings	Hamstrings, Glutes, Core	Swing kettlebell with a jump at top of motion.
85	**5 Rounds for time:**		
	(1) 10 Turkish GetUps	Shoulders, Core, Legs	Stand from floor, kettlebell overhead, controlled motion.
	(2) 15 Goblet Squats	Quads, Glutes, Core	Hold kettlebell at chest, squat, keep back straight.
	(3) 10 Burpees over Kettlebell	Full Body, Cardio	Perform burpee, jump over kettlebell.

Workout No.	Workout (Kettlebell ONLY workouts)	Main Muscle Groups	Instructions
86	**As many rounds as possible in 10 mins:**		
	(1) 20 Kettlebell Swings	Hamstrings, Glutes, Shoulders	Swing kettlebell to chest height, hinge at hips.
	(2) 15 Kettlebell Lunges (Alternating)	Quads, Glutes, Core	Step forward into lunge, hold kettlebell for balance.
	(3) 10 Renegade Rows	Back, Biceps, Core	Row kettlebells alternately in plank position.
87	**21-15-9 Reps for time:**		
	(1) Kettlebell Cleans	Shoulders, Biceps, Core	Lift kettlebell to shoulder, flip grip at top.
	(2) Kettlebell Swings	Hamstrings, Glutes, Shoulders	Swing kettlebell to chest height, hinge at hips.
	(3) Kettlebell Push Press	Shoulders, Triceps, Core	Push kettlebell overhead, lock out arms.
88	**Every minute on the minute for 25 mins:**		
	(1) 20 Kettlebell Deadlifts	Hamstrings, Glutes, Back	Lift kettlebell from ground, keep back straight.
	(2) 20 Alternating Kettlebell Lunges	Quads, Glutes, Core	Step forward into lunge, hold kettlebell for balance.
	(3) 10 Kettlebell Thrusters	Quads, Shoulders, Triceps	Squat to overhead press, one fluid motion.
89	**As many rounds as possible in 12 mins:**		
	(1) 10 Goblet Squats	Quads, Glutes, Core	Hold kettlebell at chest, squat, keep back straight.
	(2) 15 Russian Twists	Obliques, Core, Shoulders	Twist torso, touch kettlebell to ground each side.
	(3) 10 Kettlebell Snatches	Shoulders, Glutes, Hamstrings	Lift kettlebell overhead in one motion, switch hands.
90	**4 Rounds for time:**		
	(1) 10 Kettlebell Thrusters	Quads, Shoulders, Triceps	Squat to overhead press, one fluid motion.
	(2) 15 Bent Over Rows	Back, Biceps, Core	Row kettlebell to hip, switch sides.
	(3) 20 Russian Twists	Obliques, Core, Shoulders	Twist torso, touch kettlebell to ground each side.

Workout No.	Workout (Kettlebell ONLY workouts)	Main Muscle Groups	Instructions
91	**As many rounds as possible in 15 min:**		
	(1) 15 Goblet Squats	Quads, Glutes, Core	Hold kettlebell at chest, squat, keep back straight.
	(2) 12 Kettlebell Swings	Hamstrings, Glutes, Shoulders	Swing kettlebell to chest height, hinge at hips.
	(3) 10 Push Press	Shoulders, Triceps, Core	Push kettlebell overhead, lock out arms.
92	**Every minute on the minute for 20 mins:**		
	(1) 12 Kettlebell Snatches (Alternating)	Shoulders, Glutes, Hamstrings	Lift kettlebell overhead in one motion, switch hands.
	(2) 16 Russian Twists	Obliques, Core, Shoulders	Twist torso, touch kettlebell to ground each side.
93	**3 Rounds for time:**		
	(1) 15 Kettlebell Cleans	Shoulders, Biceps, Core	Lift kettlebell to shoulder, flip grip at top.
	(2) 20 Kettlebell Deadlifts	Hamstrings, Glutes, Back	Lift kettlebell from ground, keep back straight.
	(3) 15 Pushups on Kettlebell	Chest, Triceps, Shoulders	Perform pushup with hands on kettlebell.
94	**45 secs work / 15 secs rest per exercise for 4 rounds:**		
	(1) Kettlebell Thrusters	Quads, Shoulders, Triceps	Squat to overhead press, one fluid motion.
	(2) Bent Over Rows	Back, Biceps, Core	Row kettlebell to hip, switch sides.
	(3) Kettlebell Jump Swings	Hamstrings, Glutes, Core	Swing kettlebell with a jump at top of motion.
95	**5 Rounds for time:**		
	(1) 10 Turkish GetUps	Shoulders, Core, Legs	Stand from floor, kettlebell overhead, controlled motion.
	(2) 15 Goblet Squats	Quads, Glutes, Core	Hold kettlebell at chest, squat, keep back straight.
	(3) 10 Burpees over Kettlebell	Full Body, Cardio	Perform burpee, jump over kettlebell.

Workout No.	Workout (Kettlebell ONLY workouts)	Main Muscle Groups	Instructions
96	**As many rounds as possible in 10 mins:**		
	(1) 20 Kettlebell Swings	Hamstrings, Glutes, Shoulders	Swing kettlebell to chest height, hinge at hips.
	(2) 15 Kettlebell Lunges (Alternating)	Quads, Glutes, Core	Step forward into lunge, hold kettlebell for balance.
	(3) 10 Renegade Rows	Back, Biceps, Core	Row kettlebells alternately in plank position.
97	**21-15-9 Reps for time:**		
	(1) Kettlebell Cleans	Shoulders, Biceps, Core	Lift kettlebell to shoulder, flip grip at top.
	(2) Kettlebell Swings	Hamstrings, Glutes, Shoulders	Swing kettlebell to chest height, hinge at hips.
	(3) Kettlebell Push Press	Shoulders, Triceps, Core	Push kettlebell overhead, lock out arms.
98	**Every minute on the minute for 25 mins:**		
	(1) 20 Kettlebell Deadlifts	Hamstrings, Glutes, Back	Lift kettlebell from ground, keep back straight.
	(2) 20 Alternating Kettlebell Lunges	Quads, Glutes, Core	Step forward into lunge, hold kettlebell for balance.
	(3) 10 Kettlebell Thrusters	Quads, Shoulders, Triceps	Squat to overhead press, one fluid motion.
99	**As many rounds as possible in 12 mins:**		
	(1) 10 Goblet Squats	Quads, Glutes, Core	Hold kettlebell at chest, squat, keep back straight.
	(2) 15 Russian Twists	Obliques, Core, Shoulders	Twist torso, touch kettlebell to ground each side.
	(3) 10 Kettlebell Snatches	Shoulders, Glutes, Hamstrings	Lift kettlebell overhead in one motion, switch hands.
100	**4 Rounds for time:**		
	(1) 10 Kettlebell Thrusters	Quads, Shoulders, Triceps	Squat to overhead press, one fluid motion.
	(2) 15 Bent Over Rows	Back, Biceps, Core	Row kettlebell to hip, switch sides.
	(3) 20 Russian Twists	Obliques, Core, Shoulders	Twist torso, touch kettlebell to ground each side.

Workout No.	Workout (Kettlebell ONLY workouts)	Main Muscle Groups	Instructions
101	**As many rounds as possible in 15 min:**		
	(1) 15 Goblet Squats	Quads, Glutes, Core	Hold kettlebell at chest, squat, keep back straight.
	(2) 12 Kettlebell Swings	Hamstrings, Glutes, Shoulders	Swing kettlebell to chest height, hinge at hips.
	(3) 10 Push Press	Shoulders, Triceps, Core	Push kettlebell overhead, lock out arms.
102	**Every minute on the minute for 20 mins:**		
	(1) 12 Kettlebell Snatches (Alternating)	Shoulders, Glutes, Hamstrings	Lift kettlebell overhead in one motion, switch hands.
	(2) 16 Russian Twists	Obliques, Core, Shoulders	Twist torso, touch kettlebell to ground each side.
103	**3 Rounds for time:**		
	(1) 15 Kettlebell Cleans	Shoulders, Biceps, Core	Lift kettlebell to shoulder, flip grip at top.
	(2) 20 Kettlebell Deadlifts	Hamstrings, Glutes, Back	Lift kettlebell from ground, keep back straight.
	(3) 15 Pushups on Kettlebell	Chest, Triceps, Shoulders	Perform pushup with hands on kettlebell.
104	**45 secs work / 15 secs rest per exercise for 4 rounds:**		
	(1) Kettlebell Thrusters	Quads, Shoulders, Triceps	Squat to overhead press, one fluid motion.
	(2) Bent Over Rows	Back, Biceps, Core	Row kettlebell to hip, switch sides.
	(3) Kettlebell Jump Swings	Hamstrings, Glutes, Core	Swing kettlebell with a jump at top of motion.
105	**5 Rounds for time:**		
	(1) 10 Turkish GetUps	Shoulders, Core, Legs	Stand from floor, kettlebell overhead, controlled motion.
	(2) 15 Goblet Squats	Quads, Glutes, Core	Hold kettlebell at chest, squat, keep back straight.
	(3) 10 Burpees over Kettlebell	Full Body, Cardio	Perform burpee, jump over kettlebell.

Workout No.	Workout (Kettlebell ONLY workouts)		Main Muscle Groups	Instructions
106	**As many rounds as possible in 10 mins:**			
	(1)	20 Kettlebell Swings	Hamstrings, Glutes, Shoulders	Swing kettlebell to chest height, hinge at hips.
	(2)	15 Kettlebell Lunges (Alternating)	Quads, Glutes, Core	Step forward into lunge, hold kettlebell for balance.
	(3)	10 Renegade Rows	Back, Biceps, Core	Row kettlebells alternately in plank position.
107	**21-15-9 Reps for time:**			
	(1)	Kettlebell Cleans	Shoulders, Biceps, Core	Lift kettlebell to shoulder, flip grip at top.
	(2)	Kettlebell Swings	Hamstrings, Glutes, Shoulders	Swing kettlebell to chest height, hinge at hips.
	(3)	Kettlebell Push Press	Shoulders, Triceps, Core	Push kettlebell overhead, lock out arms.
108	**Every minute on the minute for 25 mins:**			
	(1)	20 Kettlebell Deadlifts	Hamstrings, Glutes, Back	Lift kettlebell from ground, keep back straight.
	(2)	20 Alternating Kettlebell Lunges	Quads, Glutes, Core	Step forward into lunge, hold kettlebell for balance.
	(3)	10 Kettlebell Thrusters	Quads, Shoulders, Triceps	Squat to overhead press, one fluid motion.
109	**As many rounds as possible in 12 mins:**			
	(1)	10 Goblet Squats	Quads, Glutes, Core	Hold kettlebell at chest, squat, keep back straight.
	(2)	15 Russian Twists	Obliques, Core, Shoulders	Twist torso, touch kettlebell to ground each side.
	(3)	10 Kettlebell Snatches	Shoulders, Glutes, Hamstrings	Lift kettlebell overhead in one motion, switch hands.
110	**4 Rounds for time:**			
	(1)	10 Kettlebell Thrusters	Quads, Shoulders, Triceps	Squat to overhead press, one fluid motion.
	(2)	15 Bent Over Rows	Back, Biceps, Core	Row kettlebell to hip, switch sides.
	(3)	20 Russian Twists	Obliques, Core, Shoulders	Twist torso, touch kettlebell to ground each side.

Workout No.	Workout (Kettlebell ONLY workouts)	Main Muscle Groups	Instructions
111	**As many rounds as possible in 15 min:**		
	(1) 15 Goblet Squats	Quads, Glutes, Core	Hold kettlebell at chest, squat, keep back straight.
	(2) 12 Kettlebell Swings	Hamstrings, Glutes, Shoulders	Swing kettlebell to chest height, hinge at hips.
	(3) 10 Push Press	Shoulders, Triceps, Core	Push kettlebell overhead, lock out arms.
112	**Every minute on the minute for 20 mins:**		
	(1) 12 Kettlebell Snatches (Alternating)	Shoulders, Glutes, Hamstrings	Lift kettlebell overhead in one motion, switch hands.
	(2) 16 Russian Twists	Obliques, Core, Shoulders	Twist torso, touch kettlebell to ground each side.
113	**3 Rounds for time:**		
	(1) 15 Kettlebell Cleans	Shoulders, Biceps, Core	Lift kettlebell to shoulder, flip grip at top.
	(2) 20 Kettlebell Deadlifts	Hamstrings, Glutes, Back	Lift kettlebell from ground, keep back straight.
	(3) 15 Pushups on Kettlebell	Chest, Triceps, Shoulders	Perform pushup with hands on kettlebell.
114	**45 secs work / 15 secs rest per exercise for 4 rounds:**		
	(1) Kettlebell Thrusters	Quads, Shoulders, Triceps	Squat to overhead press, one fluid motion.
	(2) Bent Over Rows	Back, Biceps, Core	Row kettlebell to hip, switch sides.
	(3) Kettlebell Jump Swings	Hamstrings, Glutes, Core	Swing kettlebell with a jump at top of motion.
115	**5 Rounds for time:**		
	(1) 10 Turkish GetUps	Shoulders, Core, Legs	Stand from floor, kettlebell overhead, controlled motion.
	(2) 15 Goblet Squats	Quads, Glutes, Core	Hold kettlebell at chest, squat, keep back straight.
	(3) 10 Burpees over Kettlebell	Full Body, Cardio	Perform burpee, jump over kettlebell.

Workout No.	Workout (Kettlebell ONLY workouts)	Main Muscle Groups	Instructions
116	**As many rounds as possible in 10 mins:**		
	(1) 20 Kettlebell Swings	Hamstrings, Glutes, Shoulders	Swing kettlebell to chest height, hinge at hips.
	(2) 15 Kettlebell Lunges (Alternating)	Quads, Glutes, Core	Step forward into lunge, hold kettlebell for balance.
	(3) 10 Renegade Rows	Back, Biceps, Core	Row kettlebells alternately in plank position.
117	**21-15-9 Reps for time:**		
	(1) Kettlebell Cleans	Shoulders, Biceps, Core	Lift kettlebell to shoulder, flip grip at top.
	(2) Kettlebell Swings	Hamstrings, Glutes, Shoulders	Swing kettlebell to chest height, hinge at hips.
	(3) Kettlebell Push Press	Shoulders, Triceps, Core	Push kettlebell overhead, lock out arms.
118	**Every minute on the minute for 25 mins:**		
	(1) 20 Kettlebell Deadlifts	Hamstrings, Glutes, Back	Lift kettlebell from ground, keep back straight.
	(2) 20 Alternating Kettlebell Lunges	Quads, Glutes, Core	Step forward into lunge, hold kettlebell for balance.
	(3) 10 Kettlebell Thrusters	Quads, Shoulders, Triceps	Squat to overhead press, one fluid motion.
119	**As many rounds as possible in 12 mins:**		
	(1) 10 Goblet Squats	Quads, Glutes, Core	Hold kettlebell at chest, squat, keep back straight.
	(2) 15 Russian Twists	Obliques, Core, Shoulders	Twist torso, touch kettlebell to ground each side.
	(3) 10 Kettlebell Snatches	Shoulders, Glutes, Hamstrings	Lift kettlebell overhead in one motion, switch hands.
120	**4 Rounds for time:**		
	(1) 10 Kettlebell Thrusters	Quads, Shoulders, Triceps	Squat to overhead press, one fluid motion.
	(2) 15 Bent Over Rows	Back, Biceps, Core	Row kettlebell to hip, switch sides.
	(3) 20 Russian Twists	Obliques, Core, Shoulders	Twist torso, touch kettlebell to ground each side.

Workout No.	Workout (Kettlebell ONLY workouts)	Main Muscle Groups	Instructions
121	**As many rounds as possible in 12 min:**		
	(1) 15 Goblet Squats	Quads, Glutes, Core	Hold kettlebell at chest, squat, keep back straight.
	(2) 10 Kettlebell Swings	Hamstrings, Glutes, Shoulders	Swing kettlebell to chest height, hinge at hips.
	(3) 5 Push Press	Shoulders, Triceps, Core	Push kettlebell overhead, lock out arms.
122	**Every minute on the minute for 20 mins:**		
	(1) 12 Kettlebell Snatches (Alternating)	Shoulders, Glutes, Hamstrings	Lift kettlebell overhead in one motion, switch hands.
	(2) 15 Russian Twists	Obliques, Core, Shoulders	Twist torso, touch kettlebell to ground each side.
123	**5 Rounds for time:**		
	(1) 15 Kettlebell Cleans	Shoulders, Biceps, Core	Lift kettlebell to shoulder, flip grip at top.
	(2) 20 Kettlebell Deadlifts	Hamstrings, Glutes, Back	Lift kettlebell from ground, keep back straight.
	(3) 15 Pushups on Kettlebell	Chest, Triceps, Shoulders	Perform pushup with hands on kettlebell.
124	**45 secs work / 15 secs rest per exercise for 4 rounds:**		
	(1) Kettlebell Thrusters	Quads, Shoulders, Triceps	Squat to overhead press, one fluid motion.
	(2) Bent Over Rows	Back, Biceps, Core	Row kettlebell to hip, switch sides.
	(3) Kettlebell Jump Swings	Hamstrings, Glutes, Core	Swing kettlebell with a jump at top of motion.
125	**4 Rounds for time:**		
	(1) 10 Turkish GetUps	Shoulders, Core, Legs	Stand from floor, kettlebell overhead, controlled motion.
	(2) 15 Goblet Squats	Quads, Glutes, Core	Hold kettlebell at chest, squat, keep back straight.
	(3) 10 Burpees over Kettlebell	Full Body, Cardio	Perform burpee, jump over kettlebell.

Workout No.	Workout (Kettlebell ONLY workouts)	Main Muscle Groups	Instructions
126	**As many rounds as possible in 10 mins:**		
	(1) 20 Kettlebell Swings	Hamstrings, Glutes, Shoulders	Swing kettlebell to chest height, hinge at hips.
	(2) 15 Kettlebell Lunges (Alternating)	Quads, Glutes, Core	Step forward into lunge, hold kettlebell for balance.
	(3) 10 Renegade Rows	Back, Biceps, Core	Row kettlebells alternately in plank position.
127	**21-15-9 Reps for time:**		
	(1) Kettlebell Cleans	Shoulders, Biceps, Core	Lift kettlebell to shoulder, flip grip at top.
	(2) Kettlebell Swings	Hamstrings, Glutes, Shoulders	Swing kettlebell to chest height, hinge at hips.
	(3) Kettlebell Push Press	Shoulders, Triceps, Core	Push kettlebell overhead, lock out arms.
128	**Every minute on the minute for 25 mins:**		
	(1) 20 Kettlebell Deadlifts	Hamstrings, Glutes, Back	Lift kettlebell from ground, keep back straight.
	(2) 20 Alternating Kettlebell Lunges	Quads, Glutes, Core	Step forward into lunge, hold kettlebell for balance.
	(3) 10 Kettlebell Thrusters	Quads, Shoulders, Triceps	Squat to overhead press, one fluid motion.
129	**As many rounds as possible in 12 mins:**		
	(1) 10 Goblet Squats	Quads, Glutes, Core	Hold kettlebell at chest, squat, keep back straight.
	(2) 15 Russian Twists	Obliques, Core, Shoulders	Twist torso, touch kettlebell to ground each side.
	(3) 10 Kettlebell Snatches	Shoulders, Glutes, Hamstrings	Lift kettlebell overhead in one motion, switch hands.
130	**4 Rounds for time:**		
	(1) 10 Kettlebell Thrusters	Quads, Shoulders, Triceps	Squat to overhead press, one fluid motion.
	(2) 15 Bent Over Rows	Back, Biceps, Core	Row kettlebell to hip, switch sides.
	(3) 20 Russian Twists	Obliques, Core, Shoulders	Twist torso, touch kettlebell to ground each side.

Workout No.	Workout (Kettlebell ONLY workouts)	Main Muscle Groups	Instructions
131	**As many rounds as possible in 10 min:**		
	(1) 15 Goblet Squats	Quads, Glutes, Core	Hold kettlebell at chest, squat, keep back straight.
	(2) 10 Kettlebell Swings	Hamstrings, Glutes, Shoulders	Swing kettlebell to chest height, hinge at hips.
	(3) 5 Push Press	Shoulders, Triceps, Core	Push kettlebell overhead, lock out arms.
132	**Every minute on the minute for 20 mins:**		
	(1) 12 Kettlebell Snatches (Alternating)	Shoulders, Glutes, Hamstrings	Lift kettlebell overhead in one motion, switch hands.
	(2) 15 Russian Twists	Obliques, Core, Shoulders	Twist torso, touch kettlebell to ground each side.
133	**5 Rounds for time:**		
	(1) 15 Kettlebell Cleans	Shoulders, Biceps, Core	Lift kettlebell to shoulder, flip grip at top.
	(2) 20 Kettlebell Deadlifts	Hamstrings, Glutes, Back	Lift kettlebell from ground, keep back straight.
	(3) 15 Pushups on Kettlebell	Chest, Triceps, Shoulders	Perform pushup with hands on kettlebell.
134	**45 secs work / 15 secs rest per exercise for 4 rounds:**		
	(1) Kettlebell Thrusters	Quads, Shoulders, Triceps	Squat to overhead press, one fluid motion.
	(2) Bent Over Rows	Back, Biceps, Core	Row kettlebell to hip, switch sides.
	(3) Kettlebell Jump Swings	Hamstrings, Glutes, Core	Swing kettlebell with a jump at top of motion.
135	**4 Rounds for time:**		
	(1) 10 Turkish GetUps	Shoulders, Core, Legs	Stand from floor, kettlebell overhead, controlled motion.
	(2) 15 Goblet Squats	Quads, Glutes, Core	Hold kettlebell at chest, squat, keep back straight.
	(3) 10 Burpees over Kettlebell	Full Body, Cardio	Perform burpee, jump over kettlebell.

Workout No.	Workout (Kettlebell ONLY workouts)	Main Muscle Groups	Instructions
136	**As many rounds as possible in 10 mins:**		
	(1) 20 Kettlebell Swings	Hamstrings, Glutes, Shoulders	Swing kettlebell to chest height, hinge at hips.
	(2) 15 Kettlebell Lunges (Alternating)	Quads, Glutes, Core	Step forward into lunge, hold kettlebell for balance.
	(3) 10 Renegade Rows	Back, Biceps, Core	Row kettlebells alternately in plank position.
137	**21-15-9 Reps for time:**		
	(1) Kettlebell Cleans	Shoulders, Biceps, Core	Lift kettlebell to shoulder, flip grip at top.
	(2) Kettlebell Swings	Hamstrings, Glutes, Shoulders	Swing kettlebell to chest height, hinge at hips.
	(3) Kettlebell Push Press	Shoulders, Triceps, Core	Push kettlebell overhead, lock out arms.
138	**Every minute on the minute for 25 mins:**		
	(1) 20 Kettlebell Deadlifts	Hamstrings, Glutes, Back	Lift kettlebell from ground, keep back straight.
	(2) 20 Alternating Kettlebell Lunges	Quads, Glutes, Core	Step forward into lunge, hold kettlebell for balance.
	(3) 10 Kettlebell Thrusters	Quads, Shoulders, Triceps	Squat to overhead press, one fluid motion.
139	**As many rounds as possible in 12 mins:**		
	(1) 10 Goblet Squats	Quads, Glutes, Core	Hold kettlebell at chest, squat, keep back straight.
	(2) 15 Russian Twists	Obliques, Core, Shoulders	Twist torso, touch kettlebell to ground each side.
	(3) 10 Kettlebell Snatches	Shoulders, Glutes, Hamstrings	Lift kettlebell overhead in one motion, switch hands.
140	**4 Rounds for time:**		
	(1) 10 Kettlebell Thrusters	Quads, Shoulders, Triceps	Squat to overhead press, one fluid motion.
	(2) 15 Bent Over Rows	Back, Biceps, Core	Row kettlebell to hip, switch sides.
	(3) 20 Russian Twists	Obliques, Core, Shoulders	Twist torso, touch kettlebell to ground each side.

Workout No.	Workout (Kettlebell ONLY workouts)		Main Muscle Groups	Instructions
141	**As many rounds as possible in 15 min:**			
	(1)	15 Goblet Squats	Quads, Glutes, Core	Hold kettlebell at chest, squat, keep back straight.
	(2)	10 Kettlebell Swings	Hamstrings, Glutes, Shoulders	Swing kettlebell to chest height, hinge at hips.
	(3)	5 Push Press	Shoulders, Triceps, Core	Push kettlebell overhead, lock out arms.
142	**Every minute on the minute for 20 mins:**			
	(1)	12 Kettlebell Snatches (Alternating)	Shoulders, Glutes, Hamstrings	Lift kettlebell overhead in one motion, switch hands.
	(2)	15 Russian Twists	Obliques, Core, Shoulders	Twist torso, touch kettlebell to ground each side.
143	**5 Rounds for time:**			
	(1)	15 Kettlebell Cleans	Shoulders, Biceps, Core	Lift kettlebell to shoulder, flip grip at top.
	(2)	20 Kettlebell Deadlifts	Hamstrings, Glutes, Back	Lift kettlebell from ground, keep back straight.
	(3)	15 Pushups on Kettlebell	Chest, Triceps, Shoulders	Perform pushup with hands on kettlebell.
144	**45 secs work / 15 secs rest per exercise for 4 rounds:**			
	(1)	Kettlebell Thrusters	Quads, Shoulders, Triceps	Squat to overhead press, one fluid motion.
	(2)	Bent Over Rows	Back, Biceps, Core	Row kettlebell to hip, switch sides.
	(3)	Kettlebell Jump Swings	Hamstrings, Glutes, Core	Swing kettlebell with a jump at top of motion.
145	**4 Rounds for time:**			
	(1)	10 Turkish GetUps	Shoulders, Core, Legs	Stand from floor, kettlebell overhead, controlled motion.
	(2)	15 Goblet Squats	Quads, Glutes, Core	Hold kettlebell at chest, squat, keep back straight.
	(3)	10 Burpees over Kettlebell	Full Body, Cardio	Perform burpee, jump over kettlebell.

Workout No.	Workout (Kettlebell ONLY workouts)		Main Muscle Groups	Instructions
146	As many rounds as possible in 10 mins:			
	(1)	20 Kettlebell Swings	Hamstrings, Glutes, Shoulders	Swing kettlebell to chest height, hinge at hips.
	(2)	15 Kettlebell Lunges (Alternating)	Quads, Glutes, Core	Step forward into lunge, hold kettlebell for balance.
	(3)	10 Renegade Rows	Back, Biceps, Core	Row kettlebells alternately in plank position.
147	21-15-9 Reps for time:			
	(1)	Kettlebell Cleans	Shoulders, Biceps, Core	Lift kettlebell to shoulder, flip grip at top.
	(2)	Kettlebell Swings	Hamstrings, Glutes, Shoulders	Swing kettlebell to chest height, hinge at hips.
	(3)	Kettlebell Push Press	Shoulders, Triceps, Core	Push kettlebell overhead, lock out arms.
148	Every minute on the minute for 25 mins:			
	(1)	20 Kettlebell Deadlifts	Hamstrings, Glutes, Back	Lift kettlebell from ground, keep back straight.
	(2)	20 Alternating Kettlebell Lunges	Quads, Glutes, Core	Step forward into lunge, hold kettlebell for balance.
	(3)	10 Kettlebell Thrusters	Quads, Shoulders, Triceps	Squat to overhead press, one fluid motion.
149	As many rounds as possible in 12 mins:			
	(1)	10 Goblet Squats	Quads, Glutes, Core	Hold kettlebell at chest, squat, keep back straight.
	(2)	15 Russian Twists	Obliques, Core, Shoulders	Twist torso, touch kettlebell to ground each side.
	(3)	10 Kettlebell Snatches	Shoulders, Glutes, Hamstrings	Lift kettlebell overhead in one motion, switch hands.
150	4 Rounds for time:			
	(1)	10 Kettlebell Thrusters	Quads, Shoulders, Triceps	Squat to overhead press, one fluid motion.
	(2)	15 Bent Over Rows	Back, Biceps, Core	Row kettlebell to hip, switch sides.
	(3)	20 Russian Twists	Obliques, Core, Shoulders	Twist torso, touch kettlebell to ground each side.

Part IV

150 Kettlebell + Body-Weight Workouts

Workout No.	Workout (Kettlebell & Body-Weight Workouts)	Main Muscle Groups	Instructions
	Repeat 4 times with 1-minute rest between rounds:		
1	(1) 30 seconds Kettlebell Swing	Lower Body, Core, Shoulders	Swing kettlebell between legs, thrust hips forward, raise kettlebell to shoulder height. Repeat for 30 seconds.
	(2) 30 seconds Burpees	Full Body, Core, Legs	Jump, squat down, kick back into push-up, return up. Repeat for 30 seconds.
	(3) 30 seconds Goblet Squat	Legs, Core, Glutes	Squat holding kettlebell close to chest, keep back straight. Repeat for 30 seconds.
	(4) 30 seconds High Knees	Legs, Cardio, Core	Run in place lifting knees high, maintain fast pace. Repeat for 30 seconds.
	3 Rounds for time:		
2	(1) 15 Kettlebell Clean and Press	Shoulders, Arms, Core	Clean kettlebell to shoulder, press overhead. Alternate arms. Complete 15 reps each arm.
	(2) 20 Push-Ups	Chest, Triceps, Core	Lower body to ground, push up with arms. Repeat for 20 reps.
	(3) 20 Kettlebell Goblet Squat	Legs, Glutes, Core	Squat holding kettlebell close to chest. Repeat for 20 reps.
	(4) 400-meter run	Legs, Cardio, Core	Run 400 meters at a steady pace.
	Repeat 5 times::		
3	(1) 40 seconds Kettlebell Snatch	Shoulders, Back, Core	Lift kettlebell overhead in one motion, lock arm. Alternate arms. Repeat for 40 seconds.
	(2) 20 seconds Rest		Rest for 20 seconds.
	(3) 40 seconds Mountain Climbers	Cardio, Core, Legs	Run in place in plank position, drive knees to chest. Repeat for 40 seconds.
	(4) 20 seconds Rest		Rest for 20 seconds.
	As many rounds as possible in 12 mins of:		
4	(1) 10 Kettlebell Deadlifts	Lower Back, Hamstrings, Glutes	Lift kettlebell from ground, keep back straight. Repeat for 10 reps.
	(2) 15 Box Jumps	Legs, Cardio, Core	Jump onto and off a box repeatedly. Repeat for 15 reps.
	(3) 20 Kettlebell Thrusters	Shoulders, Legs, Core	Squat to overhead press in one fluid motion. Repeat for 20 reps.
	(4) 25 Sit-Ups	Abs, Core, Hip Flexors	Perform sit-ups lying on back, hands behind head. Repeat for 25 reps.
	Repeat 4 times with 1-minute rest between rounds:		
5	(1) 30 seconds Single Arm Kettlebell Swing	Shoulders, Back, Core	Swing kettlebell with one hand, switch hands mid-air. Repeat for 30 seconds.
	(2) 30 seconds Jumping Jacks	Cardio, Legs, Core	Jump to spread legs and clap hands overhead. Repeat for 30 seconds.
	(3) 30 seconds Kettlebell Front Raise	Shoulders, Arms, Core	Lift kettlebell to shoulder height, keep arms straight. Repeat for 30 seconds.
	(4) 30 seconds Push-Ups	Chest, Triceps, Core	Lower body to ground, push up with arms. Repeat for 30 seconds.

Workout No.	Workout (Kettlebell & Body-Weight Workouts)	Main Muscle Groups	Instructions
6	**4 Rounds for time:**		
	(1) 20 Kettlebell Swings	Lower Body, Core, Shoulders	Swing kettlebell between legs, thrust hips forward. Repeat for 20 reps.
	(2) 20 Lunges	Legs, Glutes, Core	Step forward, lower hips to drop knee to ground. Repeat for 20 reps.
	(3) 15 Kettlebell Bent Over Rows	Back, Shoulders, Arms	Hinge forward, row kettlebell to hip. Repeat for 15 reps each side.
	(4) 200-meter run	Legs, Cardio, Core	Run 200 meters at a steady pace.
7	**Repeat 5 times:**		
	(1) 45 seconds Kettlebell Around the Body	Core, Shoulders, Arms	Pass kettlebell around body, maintain core control. Repeat for 45 seconds.
	(2) 15 seconds Rest		Rest for 15 seconds.
	(3) 45 seconds Burpees	Full Body, Core, Legs	Jump, squat down, kick back into push-up, return up. Repeat for 45 seconds.
	(4) 15 seconds Rest		Rest for 15 seconds.
8	**3 Rounds for time:**		
	(1) 10 Kettlebell Snatches	Shoulders, Back, Core	Lift kettlebell overhead in one motion, lock arm. Alternate arms. Complete 10 reps each arm.
	(2) 20 Air Squats	Legs, Glutes, Core	Stand, bend knees to lower body. Repeat for 20 reps.
	(3) 15 Kettlebell Deadlifts	Lower Back, Hamstrings, Glutes	Lift kettlebell from ground, keep back straight. Repeat for 15 reps.
	(4) 300-meter run	Legs, Cardio, Core	Run 300 meters at a steady pace.
9	**Repeat 8 times:**		
	(1) 20 seconds Kettlebell Jump Swing	Legs, Core, Shoulders	Explosive swing with a jump at top of motion. Repeat for 20 seconds.
	(2) 10 seconds Rest		Rest for 10 seconds.
	(3) 20 seconds Push-Up with Extension	Chest, Triceps, Core	Perform push-up, extend one arm forward. Repeat for 20 seconds.
	(4) 10 seconds Rest		Rest for 10 seconds.
10	**4 Rounds for time:**		
	(1) 15 Kettlebell Clean	Shoulders, Back, Core	Lift kettlebell to shoulder, flip grip at top. Repeat for 15 reps.
	(2) 20 V-Ups	Abs, Core, Hip Flexors	Lie back, lift legs and torso simultaneously. Repeat for 20 reps.
	(3) 20 Kettlebell Goblet Squat	Legs, Glutes, Core	Squat holding kettlebell close to chest. Repeat for 20 reps.
	(4) 250-meter run	Legs, Cardio, Core	Run 250 meters at a steady pace.

Workout No.	Workout (Kettlebell & Body-Weight Workouts)	Main Muscle Groups	Instructions
11	**3 Rounds for time:**		
	(1) 10 Kettlebell Deadlifts	Lower Back, Hamstrings, Glutes	Lift kettlebell from ground, keep back straight. Repeat for 10 reps.
	(2) 15 Push-Ups	Chest, Triceps, Core	Lower body to ground, push up with arms. Repeat for 15 reps.
	(3) 20 Kettlebell Goblet Squats	Legs, Glutes, Core	Squat holding kettlebell close to chest. Repeat for 20 reps.
	(4) 200-meter run	Legs, Cardio, Core	Run 200 meters at a steady pace.
12	**Repeat 4 times with 1-minute rest between rounds:**		
	(1) 30 seconds Kettlebell Swing	Lower Body, Core, Shoulders	Swing kettlebell between legs, thrust hips forward, raise kettlebell to shoulder height. Repeat for 30 seconds.
	(2) 30 seconds Mountain Climbers	Cardio, Core, Legs	Run in place in plank position, drive knees to chest. Repeat for 30 seconds.
	(3) 30 seconds Kettlebell Thrusters	Shoulders, Legs, Core	Squat to overhead press in one fluid motion. Repeat for 30 seconds.
	(4) 30 seconds Jumping Jacks	Cardio, Legs, Core	Jump to spread legs and clap hands overhead. Repeat for 30 seconds.
13	**3 Rounds for time:**		
	(1) 15 Kettlebell Clean and Press	Shoulders, Arms, Core	Clean kettlebell to shoulder, press overhead. Alternate arms. Complete 15 reps each arm.
	(2) 20 Air Squats	Legs, Glutes, Core	Stand, bend knees to lower body. Repeat for 20 reps.
	(3) 15 Kettlebell Bent Over Rows	Back, Shoulders, Arms	Hinge forward, row kettlebell to hip. Repeat for 15 reps each side.
	(4) 400-meter run	Legs, Cardio, Core	Run 400 meters at a steady pace.
14	**3 Rounds for time:**		
	(1) 15 Kettlebell Clean and Press	Shoulders, Back, Core	Clean kettlebell to shoulder, press overhead. Alternate arms. Complete 15 reps each arm.
	(2) 20 Air Squats		Stand, bend knees to lower body. Repeat for 20 reps.
	(3) 15 Kettlebell Bent Over Rows	Full Body, Core, Legs	Hinge forward, row kettlebell to hip. Repeat for 15 reps each side.
	(4) 400-meter run		Run 400 meters at a steady pace.
15	**4 Rounds for time:**		
	(1) 20 Kettlebell Swings	Lower Body, Core, Shoulders	Swing kettlebell between legs, thrust hips forward. Repeat for 20 reps.
	(2) 20 Lunges	Legs, Glutes, Core	Step forward, lower hips to drop knee to ground. Repeat for 20 reps.
	(3) 15 Kettlebell Shoulder Press	Shoulders, Arms, Core	Press kettlebell overhead from shoulder level. Repeat for 15 reps each side.
	(4) 200-meter run	Legs, Cardio, Core	Run 200 meters at a steady pace.

Workout No.	Workout (Kettlebell & Body-Weight Workouts)	Main Muscle Groups	Instructions
16	**Repeat 5 times:**		
	(1) 45 seconds Kettlebell Around the Body	Core, Shoulders, Arms	Pass kettlebell around body, maintain core control. Repeat for 45 seconds.
	(2) 15 seconds Rest		Rest for 15 seconds.
	(3) 45 seconds Jumping Jacks	Cardio, Legs, Core	Jump to spread legs and clap hands overhead. Repeat for 45 seconds.
	(4) 15 seconds Rest		Rest for 15 seconds.
17	**3 Rounds for time:**		
	(1) 10 Kettlebell Snatches	Shoulders, Back, Core	Lift kettlebell overhead in one motion, lock arm. Alternate arms. Complete 10 reps each arm.
	(2) 20 Push-Ups	Chest, Triceps, Core	Lower body to ground, push up with arms. Repeat for 20 reps.
	(3) 15 Kettlebell Deadlifts	Lower Back, Hamstrings, Glutes	Lift kettlebell from ground, keep back straight. Repeat for 15 reps.
	(4) 300-meter run	Legs, Cardio, Core	Run 300 meters at a steady pace.
18	**Repeat 8 times:**		
	(1) 20 seconds Kettlebell Jump Swing	Legs, Core, Shoulders	Explosive swing with a jump at top of motion. Repeat for 20 seconds.
	(2) 10 seconds Rest		Rest for 10 seconds.
	(3) 20 seconds High Knees	Legs, Cardio, Core	Run in place lifting knees high. Repeat for 20 seconds.
	(4) 10 seconds Rest		Rest for 10 seconds.
19	**4 Rounds for time:**		
	(1) 15 Kettlebell Clean	Shoulders, Back, Core	Lift kettlebell to shoulder, flip grip at top. Repeat for 15 reps.
	(2) 20 V-Ups	Abs, Core, Hip Flexors	Lie back, lift legs and torso simultaneously. Repeat for 20 reps.
	(3) 20 Kettlebell Goblet Squats	Legs, Glutes, Core	Squat holding kettlebell close to chest. Repeat for 20 reps.
	(4) 250-meter run	Legs, Cardio, Core	Run 250 meters at a steady pace.
20	**Repeat 4 times with 1-minute rest between rounds:**		
	30 seconds Kettlebell Swing	Lower Body, Core, Shoulders	Swing kettlebell between legs, thrust hips forward, raise kettlebell to shoulder height. Repeat for 30 seconds.
	30 seconds Push-Ups	Chest, Triceps, Core	Lower body to ground, push up with arms. Repeat for 30 seconds.
	30 seconds Kettlebell Goblet Squats	Legs, Glutes, Core	Squat holding kettlebell close to chest. Repeat for 30 seconds.
	30 seconds Mountain Climbers	Cardio, Core, Legs	Run in place in plank position, drive knees to chest. Repeat for 30 seconds.

Workout No.	Workout (Kettlebell & Body-Weight Workouts)	Main Muscle Groups	Instructions
21	**3 Rounds for time:**		
	(1) 10 Kettlebell Deadlifts	Lower Back, Hamstrings, Glutes	Lift kettlebell from ground, keep back straight. Repeat for 10 reps.
	(2) 15 Push-Ups	Chest, Triceps, Core	Lower body to ground, push up with arms. Repeat for 15 reps.
	(3) 20 Kettlebell Goblet Squats	Legs, Glutes, Core	Squat holding kettlebell close to chest. Repeat for 20 reps.
	(4) 200-meter run	Legs, Cardio, Core	Run 200 meters at a steady pace.
22	**Repeat 4 times with 1-minute rest between rounds:**		
	(1) 30 seconds Kettlebell Swing	Lower Body, Core, Shoulders	Swing kettlebell between legs, thrust hips forward, raise kettlebell to shoulder height. Repeat for 30 seconds.
	(2) 30 seconds Mountain Climbers	Cardio, Core, Legs	Run in place in plank position, drive knees to chest. Repeat for 30 seconds.
	(3) 30 seconds Kettlebell Thrusters	Shoulders, Legs, Core	Squat to overhead press in one fluid motion. Repeat for 30 seconds.
	(4) 30 seconds Jumping Jacks	Cardio, Legs, Core	Jump to spread legs and clap hands overhead. Repeat for 30 seconds.
23	**3 Rounds for time:**		
	(1) 15 Kettlebell Clean and Press	Shoulders, Arms, Core	Clean kettlebell to shoulder, press overhead. Alternate arms. Complete 15 reps each arm.
	(2) 20 Air Squats	Legs, Glutes, Core	Stand, bend knees to lower body. Repeat for 20 reps.
	(3) 15 Kettlebell Bent Over Rows	Back, Shoulders, Arms	Hinge forward, row kettlebell to hip. Repeat for 15 reps each side.
	(4) 400-meter run	Legs, Cardio, Core	Run 400 meters at a steady pace.
24	**Repeat 5 times:**		
	(1) 40 seconds Kettlebell Snatch	Shoulders, Back, Core	Lift kettlebell overhead in one motion, lock arm. Alternate arms. Repeat for 40 seconds.
	(2) 20 seconds Rest		Rest for 20 seconds.
	(3) 40 seconds Burpees	Full Body, Core, Legs	Jump, squat down, kick back into push-up, return up. Repeat for 40 seconds.
	(4) 20 seconds Rest		Rest for 20 seconds.
25	**4 Rounds for time:**		
	(1) 20 Kettlebell Swings	Lower Body, Core, Shoulders	Swing kettlebell between legs, thrust hips forward. Repeat for 20 reps.
	(2) 20 Lunges	Legs, Glutes, Core	Step forward, lower hips to drop knee to ground. Repeat for 20 reps.
	(3) 15 Kettlebell Shoulder Press	Shoulders, Arms, Core	Press kettlebell overhead from shoulder level. Repeat for 15 reps each side.
	(4) 200-meter run	Legs, Cardio, Core	Run 200 meters at a steady pace.

Workout No.	Workout (Kettlebell & Body-Weight Workouts)	Main Muscle Groups	Instructions
26	**Repeat 5 times:**		
	(1) 45 seconds Kettlebell Around the Body	Core, Shoulders, Arms	Pass kettlebell around body, maintain core control. Repeat for 45 seconds.
	(2) 15 seconds Rest		Rest for 15 seconds.
	(3) 45 seconds Jumping Jacks	Cardio, Legs, Core	Jump to spread legs and clap hands overhead. Repeat for 45 seconds.
	(4) 15 seconds Rest		Rest for 15 seconds.
27	**3 Rounds for time:**		
	(1) 10 Kettlebell Snatches	Shoulders, Back, Core	Lift kettlebell overhead in one motion, lock arm. Alternate arms. Complete 10 reps each arm.
	(2) 20 Push-Ups	Chest, Triceps, Core	Lower body to ground, push up with arms. Repeat for 20 reps.
	(3) 15 Kettlebell Deadlifts	Lower Back, Hamstrings, Glutes	Lift kettlebell from ground, keep back straight. Repeat for 15 reps.
	(4) 300-meter run	Legs, Cardio, Core	Run 300 meters at a steady pace.
28	**Repeat 8 times:**		
	(1) 20 seconds Kettlebell Jump Swing	Legs, Core, Shoulders	Explosive swing with a jump at top of motion. Repeat for 20 seconds.
	(2) 10 seconds Rest		Rest for 10 seconds.
	(3) 20 seconds High Knees	Legs, Cardio, Core	Run in place lifting knees high. Repeat for 20 seconds.
	(4) 10 seconds Rest		Rest for 10 seconds.
29	**4 Rounds for time:**		
	(1) 15 Kettlebell Clean	Shoulders, Back, Core	Lift kettlebell to shoulder, flip grip at top. Repeat for 15 reps.
	(2) 20 V-Ups	Abs, Core, Hip Flexors	Lie back, lift legs and torso simultaneously. Repeat for 20 reps.
	(3) 20 Kettlebell Goblet Squats	Legs, Glutes, Core	Squat holding kettlebell close to chest. Repeat for 20 reps.
	(4) 250-meter run	Legs, Cardio, Core	Run 250 meters at a steady pace.
30	**Repeat 4 times with 1-minute rest between rounds:**		
	(1) 30 seconds Kettlebell Swing	Lower Body, Core, Shoulders	Swing kettlebell between legs, thrust hips forward, raise kettlebell to shoulder height. Repeat for 30 seconds.
	(2) 30 seconds Push-Ups	Chest, Triceps, Core	Lower body to ground, push up with arms. Repeat for 30 seconds.
	(3) 30 seconds Kettlebell Goblet Squats	Legs, Glutes, Core	Squat holding kettlebell close to chest. Repeat for 30 seconds.
	(4) 30 seconds Mountain Climbers	Cardio, Core, Legs	Run in place in plank position, drive knees to chest. Repeat for 30 seconds.

Workout No.	Workout (Kettlebell & Body-Weight Workouts)	Main Muscle Groups	Instructions
31	**3 Rounds for time:**		
	(1) 10 Kettlebell Deadlifts	Lower Back, Hamstrings, Glutes	Lift kettlebell from ground, keep back straight. Repeat for 10 reps.
	(2) 15 Push-Ups	Chest, Triceps, Core	Lower body to ground, push up with arms. Repeat for 15 reps.
	(3) 20 Kettlebell Goblet Squats	Legs, Glutes, Core	Squat holding kettlebell close to chest. Repeat for 20 reps.
	(4) 200-meter run	Legs, Cardio, Core	Run 200 meters at a steady pace.
32	**Repeat 4 times with 1-minute rest between rounds:**		
	(1) 30 seconds Kettlebell Swing	Lower Body, Core, Shoulders	Swing kettlebell between legs, thrust hips forward, raise kettlebell to shoulder height. Repeat for 30 seconds.
	(2) 30 seconds Mountain Climbers	Cardio, Core, Legs	Run in place in plank position, drive knees to chest. Repeat for 30 seconds.
	(3) 30 seconds Kettlebell Thrusters	Shoulders, Legs, Core	Squat to overhead press in one fluid motion. Repeat for 30 seconds.
	(4) 30 seconds Jumping Jacks	Cardio, Legs, Core	Jump to spread legs and clap hands overhead. Repeat for 30 seconds.
33	**3 Rounds for time:**		
	(1) 15 Kettlebell Clean and Press	Shoulders, Arms, Core	Clean kettlebell to shoulder, press overhead. Alternate arms. Complete 15 reps each arm.
	(2) 20 Air Squats	Legs, Glutes, Core	Stand, bend knees to lower body. Repeat for 20 reps.
	(3) 15 Kettlebell Bent Over Rows	Back, Shoulders, Arms	Hinge forward, row kettlebell to hip. Repeat for 15 reps each side.
	(4) 400-meter run	Legs, Cardio, Core	Run 400 meters at a steady pace.
34	**Repeat 5 times:**		
	(1) 40 seconds Kettlebell Snatch	Shoulders, Back, Core	Lift kettlebell overhead in one motion, lock arm. Alternate arms. Repeat for 40 seconds.
	(2) 20 seconds Rest		Rest for 20 seconds.
	(3) 40 seconds Burpees	Full Body, Core, Legs	Jump, squat down, kick back into push-up, return up. Repeat for 40 seconds.
	(4) 20 seconds Rest		Rest for 20 seconds.
35	**4 Rounds for time:**		
	(1) 20 Kettlebell Swings	Lower Body, Core, Shoulders	Swing kettlebell between legs, thrust hips forward. Repeat for 20 reps.
	(2) 20 Lunges	Legs, Glutes, Core	Step forward, lower hips to drop knee to ground. Repeat for 20 reps.
	(3) 15 Kettlebell Shoulder Press	Shoulders, Arms, Core	Press kettlebell overhead from shoulder level. Repeat for 15 reps each side.
	(4) 200-meter run	Legs, Cardio, Core	Run 200 meters at a steady pace.

Workout No.	Workout (Kettlebell & Body-Weight Workouts)		Main Muscle Groups	Instructions
36	**Repeat 5 times:**			
	(1)	45 seconds Kettlebell Around the Body	Core, Shoulders, Arms	Pass kettlebell around body, maintain core control. Repeat for 45 seconds.
	(2)	15 seconds Rest		Rest for 15 seconds.
	(3)	45 seconds Jumping Jacks	Cardio, Legs, Core	Jump to spread legs and clap hands overhead. Repeat for 45 seconds.
	(4)	15 seconds Rest		Rest for 15 seconds.
37	**3 Rounds for time:**			
	(1)	10 Kettlebell Snatches	Shoulders, Back, Core	Lift kettlebell overhead in one motion, lock arm. Alternate arms. Complete 10 reps each arm.
	(2)	20 Push-Ups	Chest, Triceps, Core	Lower body to ground, push up with arms. Repeat for 20 reps.
	(3)	15 Kettlebell Deadlifts	Lower Back, Hamstrings, Glutes	Lift kettlebell from ground, keep back straight. Repeat for 15 reps.
	(4)	300-meter run	Legs, Cardio, Core	Run 300 meters at a steady pace.
38	**Repeat 8 times:**			
	(1)	20 seconds Kettlebell Jump Swing	Legs, Core, Shoulders	Explosive swing with a jump at top of motion. Repeat for 20 seconds.
	(2)	10 seconds Rest		Rest for 10 seconds.
	(3)	20 seconds High Knees	Legs, Cardio, Core	Run in place lifting knees high. Repeat for 20 seconds.
	(4)	10 seconds Rest		Rest for 10 seconds.
39	**4 Rounds for time:**			
	(1)	15 Kettlebell Clean	Shoulders, Back, Core	Lift kettlebell to shoulder, flip grip at top. Repeat for 15 reps.
	(2)	20 V-Ups	Abs, Core, Hip Flexors	Lie back, lift legs and torso simultaneously. Repeat for 20 reps.
	(3)	20 Kettlebell Goblet Squats	Legs, Glutes, Core	Squat holding kettlebell close to chest. Repeat for 20 reps.
	(4)	250-meter run	Legs, Cardio, Core	Run 250 meters at a steady pace.
40	**Repeat 4 times with 1-minute rest between rounds:**			
	(1)	30 seconds Kettlebell Swing	Lower Body, Core, Shoulders	Swing kettlebell between legs, thrust hips forward, raise kettlebell to shoulder height. Repeat for 30 seconds.
	(2)	30 seconds Push-Ups	Chest, Triceps, Core	Lower body to ground, push up with arms. Repeat for 30 seconds.
	(3)	30 seconds Kettlebell Goblet Squats	Legs, Glutes, Core	Squat holding kettlebell close to chest. Repeat for 30 seconds.
	(4)	30 seconds Mountain Climbers	Cardio, Core, Legs	Run in place in plank position, drive knees to chest. Repeat for 30 seconds.

Workout No.	Workout (Kettlebell & Body-Weight Workouts)	Main Muscle Groups	Instructions
41	**3 Rounds for time:**		
	(1) 10 Kettlebell Deadlifts	Lower Back, Hamstrings, Glutes	Lift kettlebell from ground, keep back straight. Repeat for 10 reps.
	(2) 15 Push-Ups	Chest, Triceps, Core	Lower body to ground, push up with arms. Repeat for 15 reps.
	(3) 20 Kettlebell Goblet Squats	Legs, Glutes, Core	Squat holding kettlebell close to chest. Repeat for 20 reps.
	(4) 200-meter run	Legs, Cardio, Core	Run 200 meters at a steady pace.
42	**Repeat 4 times with 1-minute rest between rounds:**		
	(1) 30 seconds Kettlebell Swing	Lower Body, Core, Shoulders	Swing kettlebell between legs, thrust hips forward, raise kettlebell to shoulder height. Repeat for 30 seconds.
	(2) 30 seconds Mountain Climbers	Cardio, Core, Legs	Run in place in plank position, drive knees to chest. Repeat for 30 seconds.
	(3) 30 seconds Kettlebell Thrusters	Shoulders, Legs, Core	Squat to overhead press in one fluid motion. Repeat for 30 seconds.
	(4) 30 seconds Jumping Jacks	Cardio, Legs, Core	Jump to spread legs and clap hands overhead. Repeat for 30 seconds.
43	**3 Rounds for time:**		
	(1) 15 Kettlebell Clean and Press	Shoulders, Arms, Core	Clean kettlebell to shoulder, press overhead. Alternate arms. Complete 15 reps each arm.
	(2) 20 Air Squats	Legs, Glutes, Core	Stand, bend knees to lower body. Repeat for 20 reps.
	(3) 15 Kettlebell Bent Over Rows	Back, Shoulders, Arms	Hinge forward, row kettlebell to hip. Repeat for 15 reps each side.
	(4) 400-meter run	Legs, Cardio, Core	Run 400 meters at a steady pace.
44	**Repeat 5 times:**		
	(1) 40 seconds Kettlebell Snatch	Shoulders, Back, Core	Lift kettlebell overhead in one motion, lock arm. Alternate arms. Repeat for 40 seconds.
	(2) 20 seconds Rest		Rest for 20 seconds.
	(3) 40 seconds Burpees	Full Body, Core, Legs	Jump, squat down, kick back into push-up, return up. Repeat for 40 seconds.
	(4) 20 seconds Rest		Rest for 20 seconds.
45	**4 Rounds for time:**		
	(1) 20 Kettlebell Swings	Lower Body, Core, Shoulders	Swing kettlebell between legs, thrust hips forward. Repeat for 20 reps.
	(2) 20 Lunges	Legs, Glutes, Core	Step forward, lower hips to drop knee to ground. Repeat for 20 reps.
	(3) 15 Kettlebell Shoulder Press	Shoulders, Arms, Core	Press kettlebell overhead from shoulder level. Repeat for 15 reps each side.
	(4) 200-meter run	Legs, Cardio, Core	Run 200 meters at a steady pace.

Workout No.	Workout (Kettlebell & Body-Weight Workouts)		Main Muscle Groups	Instructions
46	**Repeat 5 times:**			
	(1)	45 seconds Kettlebell Around the Body	Core, Shoulders, Arms	Pass kettlebell around body, maintain core control. Repeat for 45 seconds.
	(2)	15 seconds Rest		Rest for 15 seconds.
	(3)	45 seconds Jumping Jacks	Cardio, Legs, Core	Jump to spread legs and clap hands overhead. Repeat for 45 seconds.
	(4)	15 seconds Rest		Rest for 15 seconds.
47	**3 Rounds for time:**			
	(1)	10 Kettlebell Snatches	Shoulders, Back, Core	Lift kettlebell overhead in one motion, lock arm. Alternate arms. Complete 10 reps each arm.
	(2)	20 Push-Ups	Chest, Triceps, Core	Lower body to ground, push up with arms. Repeat for 20 reps.
	(3)	15 Kettlebell Deadlifts	Lower Back, Hamstrings, Glutes	Lift kettlebell from ground, keep back straight. Repeat for 15 reps.
	(4)	300-meter run	Legs, Cardio, Core	Run 300 meters at a steady pace.
48	**Repeat 8 times:**			
	(1)	20 seconds Kettlebell Jump Swing	Legs, Core, Shoulders	Explosive swing with a jump at top of motion. Repeat for 20 seconds.
	(2)	10 seconds Rest		Rest for 10 seconds.
	(3)	20 seconds High Knees	Legs, Cardio, Core	Run in place lifting knees high. Repeat for 20 seconds.
	(4)	10 seconds Rest		Rest for 10 seconds.
49	**4 Rounds for time:**			
	(1)	15 Kettlebell Clean	Shoulders, Back, Core	Lift kettlebell to shoulder, flip grip at top. Repeat for 15 reps.
	(2)	20 V-Ups	Abs, Core, Hip Flexors	Lie back, lift legs and torso simultaneously. Repeat for 20 reps.
	(3)	20 Kettlebell Goblet Squats	Legs, Glutes, Core	Squat holding kettlebell close to chest. Repeat for 20 reps.
	(4)	250-meter run	Legs, Cardio, Core	Run 250 meters at a steady pace.
50	**Repeat 4 times with 1-minute rest between rounds:**			
	(1)	30 seconds Kettlebell Swing	Lower Body, Core, Shoulders	Swing kettlebell between legs, thrust hips forward, raise kettlebell to shoulder height. Repeat for 30 seconds.
	(2)	30 seconds Push-Ups	Chest, Triceps, Core	Lower body to ground, push up with arms. Repeat for 30 seconds.
	(3)	30 seconds Kettlebell Goblet Squats	Legs, Glutes, Core	Squat holding kettlebell close to chest. Repeat for 30 seconds.
	(4)	30 seconds Mountain Climbers	Cardio, Core, Legs	Run in place in plank position, drive knees to chest. Repeat for 30 seconds.

Workout No.	Workout (Kettlebell & Body-Weight Workouts)	Main Muscle Groups	Instructions
51	**3 Rounds for time:**		
	(1) 10 Kettlebell Deadlifts	Lower Back, Hamstrings, Glutes	Lift kettlebell from ground, keep back straight. Repeat for 10 reps.
	(2) 15 Push-Ups	Chest, Triceps, Core	Lower body to ground, push up with arms. Repeat for 15 reps.
	(3) 20 Kettlebell Goblet Squats	Legs, Glutes, Core	Squat holding kettlebell close to chest. Repeat for 20 reps.
	(4) 200-meter run	Legs, Cardio, Core	Run 200 meters at a steady pace.
52	**Repeat 4 times with 1-minute rest between rounds:**		
	(1) 30 seconds Kettlebell Swing	Lower Body, Core, Shoulders	Swing kettlebell between legs, thrust hips forward, raise kettlebell to shoulder height. Repeat for 30 seconds.
	(2) 30 seconds Mountain Climbers	Cardio, Core, Legs	Run in place in plank position, drive knees to chest. Repeat for 30 seconds.
	(3) 30 seconds Kettlebell Thrusters	Shoulders, Legs, Core	Squat to overhead press in one fluid motion. Repeat for 30 seconds.
	(4) 30 seconds Jumping Jacks	Cardio, Legs, Core	Jump to spread legs and clap hands overhead. Repeat for 30 seconds.
53	**3 Rounds for time:**		
	(1) 15 Kettlebell Clean and Press	Shoulders, Arms, Core	Clean kettlebell to shoulder, press overhead. Alternate arms. Complete 15 reps each arm.
	(2) 20 Air Squats	Legs, Glutes, Core	Stand, bend knees to lower body. Repeat for 20 reps.
	(3) 15 Kettlebell Bent Over Rows	Back, Shoulders, Arms	Hinge forward, row kettlebell to hip. Repeat for 15 reps each side.
	(4) 400-meter run	Legs, Cardio, Core	Run 400 meters at a steady pace.
54	**Repeat 5 times:**		
	(1) 40 seconds Kettlebell Snatch	Shoulders, Back, Core	Lift kettlebell overhead in one motion, lock arm. Alternate arms. Repeat for 40 seconds.
	(2) 20 seconds Rest		Rest for 20 seconds.
	(3) 40 seconds Burpees	Full Body, Core, Legs	Jump, squat down, kick back into push-up, return up. Repeat for 40 seconds.
	(4) 20 seconds Rest		Rest for 20 seconds.
55	**4 Rounds for time:**		
	(1) 20 Kettlebell Swings	Lower Body, Core, Shoulders	Swing kettlebell between legs, thrust hips forward. Repeat for 20 reps.
	(2) 20 Lunges	Legs, Glutes, Core	Step forward, lower hips to drop knee to ground. Repeat for 20 reps.
	(3) 15 Kettlebell Shoulder Press	Shoulders, Arms, Core	Press kettlebell overhead from shoulder level. Repeat for 15 reps each side.
	(4) 200-meter run	Legs, Cardio, Core	Run 200 meters at a steady pace.

Workout No.	Workout (Kettlebell & Body-Weight Workouts)		Main Muscle Groups	Instructions
56	Repeat 5 times:			
	(1)	45 seconds Kettlebell Around the Body	Core, Shoulders, Arms	Pass kettlebell around body, maintain core control. Repeat for 45 seconds.
	(2)	15 seconds Rest		Rest for 15 seconds.
	(3)	45 seconds Jumping Jacks	Cardio, Legs, Core	Jump to spread legs and clap hands overhead. Repeat for 45 seconds.
	(4)	15 seconds Rest		Rest for 15 seconds.
57	3 Rounds for time:			
	(1)	10 Kettlebell Snatches	Shoulders, Back, Core	Lift kettlebell overhead in one motion, lock arm. Alternate arms. Complete 10 reps each arm.
	(2)	20 Push-Ups	Chest, Triceps, Core	Lower body to ground, push up with arms. Repeat for 20 reps.
	(3)	15 Kettlebell Deadlifts	Lower Back, Hamstrings, Glutes	Lift kettlebell from ground, keep back straight. Repeat for 15 reps.
	(4)	300-meter run	Legs, Cardio, Core	Run 300 meters at a steady pace.
58	Repeat 8 times:			
	(1)	20 seconds Kettlebell Jump Swing	Legs, Core, Shoulders	Explosive swing with a jump at top of motion. Repeat for 20 seconds.
	(2)	10 seconds Rest		Rest for 10 seconds.
	(3)	20 seconds High Knees	Legs, Cardio, Core	Run in place lifting knees high. Repeat for 20 seconds.
	(4)	10 seconds Rest		Rest for 10 seconds.
59	4 Rounds for time:			
	(1)	15 Kettlebell Clean	Shoulders, Back, Core	Lift kettlebell to shoulder, flip grip at top. Repeat for 15 reps.
	(2)	20 V-Ups	Abs, Core, Hip Flexors	Lie back, lift legs and torso simultaneously. Repeat for 20 reps.
	(3)	20 Kettlebell Goblet Squats	Legs, Glutes, Core	Squat holding kettlebell close to chest. Repeat for 20 reps.
	(4)	250-meter run	Legs, Cardio, Core	Run 250 meters at a steady pace.
60	Repeat 4 times with 1-minute rest between rounds:			
	(1)	30 seconds Kettlebell Swing	Lower Body, Core, Shoulders	Swing kettlebell between legs, thrust hips forward, raise kettlebell to shoulder height. Repeat for 30 seconds.
	(2)	30 seconds Push-Ups	Chest, Triceps, Core	Lower body to ground, push up with arms. Repeat for 30 seconds.
	(3)	30 seconds Kettlebell Goblet Squats	Legs, Glutes, Core	Squat holding kettlebell close to chest. Repeat for 30 seconds.
	(4)	30 seconds Mountain Climbers	Cardio, Core, Legs	Run in place in plank position, drive knees to chest. Repeat for 30 seconds.

Workout No.	Workout (Kettlebell & Body-Weight Workouts)	Main Muscle Groups	Instructions
61	**3 Rounds for time:**		
	(1) 10 Kettlebell Deadlifts	Lower Back, Hamstrings, Glutes	Lift kettlebell from ground, keep back straight. Repeat for 10 reps.
	(2) 15 Push-Ups	Chest, Triceps, Core	Lower body to ground, push up with arms. Repeat for 15 reps.
	(3) 20 Kettlebell Goblet Squats	Legs, Glutes, Core	Squat holding kettlebell close to chest. Repeat for 20 reps.
	(4) 200-meter run	Legs, Cardio, Core	Run 200 meters at a steady pace.
62	**Repeat 4 times with 1-minute rest between rounds:**		
	(1) 30 seconds Kettlebell Swing	Lower Body, Core, Shoulders	Swing kettlebell between legs, thrust hips forward, raise kettlebell to shoulder height. Repeat for 30 seconds.
	(2) 30 seconds Mountain Climbers	Cardio, Core, Legs	Run in place in plank position, drive knees to chest. Repeat for 30 seconds.
	(3) 30 seconds Kettlebell Thrusters	Shoulders, Legs, Core	Squat to overhead press in one fluid motion. Repeat for 30 seconds.
	(4) 30 seconds Jumping Jacks	Cardio, Legs, Core	Jump to spread legs and clap hands overhead. Repeat for 30 seconds.
63	**3 Rounds for time:**		
	(1) 15 Kettlebell Clean and Press	Shoulders, Arms, Core	Clean kettlebell to shoulder, press overhead. Alternate arms. Complete 15 reps each arm.
	(2) 20 Air Squats	Legs, Glutes, Core	Stand, bend knees to lower body. Repeat for 20 reps.
	(3) 15 Kettlebell Bent Over Rows	Back, Shoulders, Arms	Hinge forward, row kettlebell to hip. Repeat for 15 reps each side.
	(4) 400-meter run	Legs, Cardio, Core	Run 400 meters at a steady pace.
64	**Repeat 5 times:**		
	(1) 40 seconds Kettlebell Snatch	Shoulders, Back, Core	Lift kettlebell overhead in one motion, lock arm. Alternate arms. Repeat for 40 seconds.
	(2) 20 seconds Rest		Rest for 20 seconds.
	(3) 40 seconds Burpees	Full Body, Core, Legs	Jump, squat down, kick back into push-up, return up. Repeat for 40 seconds.
	(4) 20 seconds Rest		Rest for 20 seconds.
65	**4 Rounds for time:**		
	(1) 20 Kettlebell Swings	Lower Body, Core, Shoulders	Swing kettlebell between legs, thrust hips forward. Repeat for 20 reps.
	(2) 20 Lunges	Legs, Glutes, Core	Step forward, lower hips to drop knee to ground. Repeat for 20 reps.
	(3) 15 Kettlebell Shoulder Press	Shoulders, Arms, Core	Press kettlebell overhead from shoulder level. Repeat for 15 reps each side.
	(4) 200-meter run	Legs, Cardio, Core	Run 200 meters at a steady pace.

Workout No.	Workout (Kettlebell & Body-Weight Workouts)	Main Muscle Groups	Instructions
66	**Repeat 5 times:**		
	(1) 45 seconds Kettlebell Around the Body	Core, Shoulders, Arms	Pass kettlebell around body, maintain core control. Repeat for 45 seconds.
	(2) 15 seconds Rest		Rest for 15 seconds.
	(3) 45 seconds Jumping Jacks	Cardio, Legs, Core	Jump to spread legs and clap hands overhead. Repeat for 45 seconds.
	(4) 15 seconds Rest		Rest for 15 seconds.
67	**3 Rounds for time:**		
	(1) 10 Kettlebell Snatches	Shoulders, Back, Core	Lift kettlebell overhead in one motion, lock arm. Alternate arms. Complete 10 reps each arm.
	(2) 20 Push-Ups	Chest, Triceps, Core	Lower body to ground, push up with arms. Repeat for 20 reps.
	(3) 15 Kettlebell Deadlifts	Lower Back, Hamstrings, Glutes	Lift kettlebell from ground, keep back straight. Repeat for 15 reps.
	(4) 300-meter run	Legs, Cardio, Core	Run 300 meters at a steady pace.
68	**Repeat 8 times:**		
	(1) 20 seconds Kettlebell Jump Swing	Legs, Core, Shoulders	Explosive swing with a jump at top of motion. Repeat for 20 seconds.
	(2) 10 seconds Rest		Rest for 10 seconds.
	(3) 20 seconds High Knees	Legs, Cardio, Core	Run in place lifting knees high. Repeat for 20 seconds.
	(4) 10 seconds Rest		Rest for 10 seconds.
69	**4 Rounds for time:**		
	(1) 15 Kettlebell Clean	Shoulders, Back, Core	Lift kettlebell to shoulder, flip grip at top. Repeat for 15 reps.
	(2) 20 V-Ups	Abs, Core, Hip Flexors	Lie back, lift legs and torso simultaneously. Repeat for 20 reps.
	(3) 20 Kettlebell Goblet Squats	Legs, Glutes, Core	Squat holding kettlebell close to chest. Repeat for 20 reps.
	(4) 250-meter run	Legs, Cardio, Core	Run 250 meters at a steady pace.
70	**Repeat 4 times with 1-minute rest between rounds:**		
	(1) 30 seconds Kettlebell Swing	Lower Body, Core, Shoulders	Swing kettlebell between legs, thrust hips forward, raise kettlebell to shoulder height. Repeat for 30 seconds.
	(2) 30 seconds Push-Ups	Chest, Triceps, Core	Lower body to ground, push up with arms. Repeat for 30 seconds.
	(3) 30 seconds Kettlebell Goblet Squats	Legs, Glutes, Core	Squat holding kettlebell close to chest. Repeat for 30 seconds.
	(4) 30 seconds Mountain Climbers	Cardio, Core, Legs	Run in place in plank position, drive knees to chest. Repeat for 30 seconds.

Workout No.	Workout (Kettlebell & Body-Weight Workouts)	Main Muscle Groups	Instructions
	3 Rounds for time:		
71	(1) 10 Kettlebell Deadlifts	Lower Back, Hamstrings, Glutes	Lift kettlebell from ground, keep back straight. Repeat for 10 reps.
	(2) 15 Push-Ups	Chest, Triceps, Core	Lower body to ground, push up with arms. Repeat for 15 reps.
	(3) 20 Kettlebell Goblet Squats	Legs, Glutes, Core	Squat holding kettlebell close to chest. Repeat for 20 reps.
	(4) 200-meter run	Legs, Cardio, Core	Run 200 meters at a steady pace.
	Repeat 4 times with 1-minute rest between rounds:		
72	(1) 30 seconds Kettlebell Swing	Lower Body, Core, Shoulders	Swing kettlebell between legs, thrust hips forward, raise kettlebell to shoulder height. Repeat for 30 seconds.
	(2) 30 seconds Mountain Climbers	Cardio, Core, Legs	Run in place in plank position, drive knees to chest. Repeat for 30 seconds.
	(3) 30 seconds Kettlebell Thrusters	Shoulders, Legs, Core	Squat to overhead press in one fluid motion. Repeat for 30 seconds.
	(4) 30 seconds Jumping Jacks	Cardio, Legs, Core	Jump to spread legs and clap hands overhead. Repeat for 30 seconds.
	3 Rounds for time:		
73	(1) 15 Kettlebell Clean and Press	Shoulders, Arms, Core	Clean kettlebell to shoulder, press overhead. Alternate arms. Complete 15 reps each arm.
	(2) 20 Air Squats	Legs, Glutes, Core	Stand, bend knees to lower body. Repeat for 20 reps.
	(3) 15 Kettlebell Bent Over Rows	Back, Shoulders, Arms	Hinge forward, row kettlebell to hip. Repeat for 15 reps each side.
	(4) 400-meter run	Legs, Cardio, Core	Run 400 meters at a steady pace.
	Repeat 5 times:		
74	(1) 40 seconds Kettlebell Snatch	Shoulders, Back, Core	Lift kettlebell overhead in one motion, lock arm. Alternate arms. Repeat for 40 seconds.
	(2) 20 seconds Rest		Rest for 20 seconds.
	(3) 40 seconds Burpees	Full Body, Core, Legs	Jump, squat down, kick back into push-up, return up. Repeat for 40 seconds.
	(4) 20 seconds Rest		Rest for 20 seconds.
	4 Rounds for time:		
75	(1) 20 Kettlebell Swings	Lower Body, Core, Shoulders	Swing kettlebell between legs, thrust hips forward. Repeat for 20 reps.
	(2) 20 Lunges	Legs, Glutes, Core	Step forward, lower hips to drop knee to ground. Repeat for 20 reps.
	(3) 15 Kettlebell Shoulder Press	Shoulders, Arms, Core	Press kettlebell overhead from shoulder level. Repeat for 15 reps each side.
	(4) 200-meter run	Legs, Cardio, Core	Run 200 meters at a steady pace.

Workout No.	Workout (Kettlebell & Body-Weight Workouts)	Main Muscle Groups	Instructions
76	**Repeat 5 times:**		
	(1) 45 seconds Kettlebell Around the Body	Core, Shoulders, Arms	Pass kettlebell around body, maintain core control. Repeat for 45 seconds.
	(2) 15 seconds Rest		Rest for 15 seconds.
	(3) 45 seconds Jumping Jacks	Cardio, Legs, Core	Jump to spread legs and clap hands overhead. Repeat for 45 seconds.
	(4) 15 seconds Rest		Rest for 15 seconds.
77	**3 Rounds for time:**		
	(1) 10 Kettlebell Snatches	Shoulders, Back, Core	Lift kettlebell overhead in one motion, lock arm. Alternate arms. Complete 10 reps each arm.
	(2) 20 Push-Ups	Chest, Triceps, Core	Lower body to ground, push up with arms. Repeat for 20 reps.
	(3) 15 Kettlebell Deadlifts	Lower Back, Hamstrings, Glutes	Lift kettlebell from ground, keep back straight. Repeat for 15 reps.
	(4) 300-meter run	Legs, Cardio, Core	Run 300 meters at a steady pace.
78	**Repeat 8 times:**		
	(1) 20 seconds Kettlebell Jump Swing	Legs, Core, Shoulders	Explosive swing with a jump at top of motion. Repeat for 20 seconds.
	(2) 10 seconds Rest		Rest for 10 seconds.
	(3) 20 seconds High Knees	Legs, Cardio, Core	Run in place lifting knees high. Repeat for 20 seconds.
	(4) 10 seconds Rest		Rest for 10 seconds.
79	**4 Rounds for time:**		
	(1) 15 Kettlebell Clean	Shoulders, Back, Core	Lift kettlebell to shoulder, flip grip at top. Repeat for 15 reps.
	(2) 20 V-Ups	Abs, Core, Hip Flexors	Lie back, lift legs and torso simultaneously. Repeat for 20 reps.
	(3) 20 Kettlebell Goblet Squats	Legs, Glutes, Core	Squat holding kettlebell close to chest. Repeat for 20 reps.
	(4) 250-meter run	Legs, Cardio, Core	Run 250 meters at a steady pace.
80	**Repeat 4 times with 1-minute rest between rounds:**		
	(1) 30 seconds Kettlebell Swing	Lower Body, Core, Shoulders	Swing kettlebell between legs, thrust hips forward, raise kettlebell to shoulder height. Repeat for 30 seconds.
	(2) 30 seconds Push-Ups	Chest, Triceps, Core	Lower body to ground, push up with arms. Repeat for 30 seconds.
	(3) 30 seconds Kettlebell Goblet Squats	Legs, Glutes, Core	Squat holding kettlebell close to chest. Repeat for 30 seconds.
	(4) 30 seconds Mountain Climbers	Cardio, Core, Legs	Run in place in plank position, drive knees to chest. Repeat for 30 seconds.

Workout No.	Workout (Kettlebell & Body-Weight Workouts)	Main Muscle Groups	Instructions
81	**4 Rounds for time:**		
	(1) 15 Kettlebell Deadlifts	Lower Back, Hamstrings, Glutes	Lift kettlebell from ground, keep back straight. Repeat for 15 reps.
	(2) 20 Push-Ups	Chest, Triceps, Core	Lower body to ground, push up with arms. Repeat for 20 reps.
	(3) 25 Kettlebell Goblet Squats	Legs, Glutes, Core	Squat holding kettlebell close to chest. Repeat for 25 reps.
	(4) 400-meter run	Legs, Cardio, Core	Run 400 meters at a steady pace.
82	**Repeat 4 times with 1-minute rest between rounds:**		
	(1) 30 seconds Kettlebell Swing	Lower Body, Core, Shoulders	Swing kettlebell between legs, thrust hips forward, raise kettlebell to shoulder height. Repeat for 30 seconds.
	(2) 30 seconds Mountain Climbers	Cardio, Core, Legs	Run in place in plank position, drive knees to chest. Repeat for 30 seconds.
	(3) 30 seconds Kettlebell Thrusters	Shoulders, Legs, Core	Squat to overhead press in one fluid motion. Repeat for 30 seconds.
	(4) 30 seconds Jumping Jacks	Cardio, Legs, Core	Jump to spread legs and clap hands overhead. Repeat for 30 seconds.
83	**3 Rounds for time:**		
	(1) 12 Kettlebell Clean and Press	Shoulders, Arms, Core	Clean kettlebell to shoulder, press overhead. Alternate arms. Complete 12 reps each arm.
	(2) 20 Air Squats	Legs, Glutes, Core	Stand, bend knees to lower body. Repeat for 20 reps.
	(3) 15 Kettlebell Bent Over Rows	Back, Shoulders, Arms	Hinge forward, row kettlebell to hip. Repeat for 15 reps each side.
	(4) 500-meter run	Legs, Cardio, Core	Run 500 meters at a steady pace.
84	**Repeat 5 times:**		
	(1) 40 seconds Kettlebell Snatch	Shoulders, Back, Core	Lift kettlebell overhead in one motion, lock arm. Alternate arms. Repeat for 40 seconds.
	(2) 20 seconds Rest		Rest for 20 seconds.
	(3) 40 seconds Burpees	Full Body, Core, Legs	Jump, squat down, kick back into push-up, return up. Repeat for 40 seconds.
	(4) 20 seconds Rest		Rest for 20 seconds.
85	**4 Rounds for time:**		
	(1) 20 Kettlebell Swings	Lower Body, Core, Shoulders	Swing kettlebell between legs, thrust hips forward. Repeat for 20 reps.
	(2) 20 Lunges	Legs, Glutes, Core	Step forward, lower hips to drop knee to ground. Repeat for 20 reps.
	(3) 15 Kettlebell Shoulder Press	Shoulders, Arms, Core	Press kettlebell overhead from shoulder level. Repeat for 15 reps each side.
	(4) 300-meter run	Legs, Cardio, Core	Run 300 meters at a steady pace.

Workout No.	Workout (Kettlebell & Body-Weight Workouts)	Main Muscle Groups	Instructions
86	**Repeat 5 times:**		
	(1) 45 seconds Kettlebell Around the Body	Core, Shoulders, Arms	Pass kettlebell around body, maintain core control. Repeat for 45 seconds.
	(2) 15 seconds Rest		Rest for 15 seconds.
	(3) 45 seconds Jumping Jacks	Cardio, Legs, Core	Jump to spread legs and clap hands overhead. Repeat for 45 seconds.
	(4) 15 seconds Rest		Rest for 15 seconds.
87	**3 Rounds for time:**		
	(1) 10 Kettlebell Snatches	Shoulders, Back, Core	Lift kettlebell overhead in one motion, lock arm. Alternate arms. Complete 10 reps each arm.
	(2) 20 Push-Ups	Chest, Triceps, Core	Lower body to ground, push up with arms. Repeat for 20 reps.
	(3) 15 Kettlebell Deadlifts	Lower Back, Hamstrings, Glutes	Lift kettlebell from ground, keep back straight. Repeat for 15 reps.
	(4) 300-meter run	Legs, Cardio, Core	Run 300 meters at a steady pace.
88	**Repeat 8 times:**		
	(1) 20 seconds Kettlebell Jump Swing	Legs, Core, Shoulders	Explosive swing with a jump at top of motion. Repeat for 20 seconds.
	(2) 10 seconds Rest		Rest for 10 seconds.
	(3) 20 seconds High Knees	Legs, Cardio, Core	Run in place lifting knees high. Repeat for 20 seconds.
	(4) 10 seconds Rest		Rest for 10 seconds.
89	**4 Rounds for time:**		
	(1) 15 Kettlebell Clean	Shoulders, Back, Core	Lift kettlebell to shoulder, flip grip at top. Repeat for 15 reps.
	(2) 20 V-Ups	Abs, Core, Hip Flexors	Lie back, lift legs and torso simultaneously. Repeat for 20 reps.
	(3) 20 Kettlebell Goblet Squats	Legs, Glutes, Core	Squat holding kettlebell close to chest. Repeat for 20 reps.
	(4) 250-meter run	Legs, Cardio, Core	Run 250 meters at a steady pace.
90	**Repeat 4 times with 1-minute rest between rounds:**		
	(1) 30 seconds Kettlebell Swing	Lower Body, Core, Shoulders	Swing kettlebell between legs, thrust hips forward, raise kettlebell to shoulder height. Repeat for 30 seconds.
	(2) 30 seconds Push-Ups	Chest, Triceps, Core	Lower body to ground, push up with arms. Repeat for 30 seconds.
	(3) 30 seconds Kettlebell Goblet Squats	Legs, Glutes, Core	Squat holding kettlebell close to chest. Repeat for 30 seconds.
	(4) 30 seconds Mountain Climbers	Cardio, Core, Legs	Run in place in plank position, drive knees to chest. Repeat for 30 seconds.

Workout No.	Workout (Kettlebell & Body-Weight Workouts)	Main Muscle Groups	Instructions
	4 Rounds for time:		
91	(1) 15 Kettlebell Deadlifts	Lower Back, Hamstrings, Glutes	Lift kettlebell from ground, keep back straight. Repeat for 15 reps.
	(2) 20 Push-Ups	Chest, Triceps, Core	Lower body to ground, push up with arms. Repeat for 20 reps.
	(3) 25 Kettlebell Goblet Squats	Legs, Glutes, Core	Squat holding kettlebell close to chest. Repeat for 25 reps.
	(4) 400-meter run	Legs, Cardio, Core	Run 400 meters at a steady pace.
	Repeat 4 times with 1-minute rest between rounds:		
92	(1) 30 seconds Kettlebell Swing	Lower Body, Core, Shoulders	Swing kettlebell between legs, thrust hips forward, raise kettlebell to shoulder height. Repeat for 30 seconds.
	(2) 30 seconds Mountain Climbers	Cardio, Core, Legs	Run in place in plank position, drive knees to chest. Repeat for 30 seconds.
	(3) 30 seconds Kettlebell Thrusters	Shoulders, Legs, Core	Squat to overhead press in one fluid motion. Repeat for 30 seconds.
	(4) 30 seconds Jumping Jacks	Cardio, Legs, Core	Jump to spread legs and clap hands overhead. Repeat for 30 seconds.
	3 Rounds for time:		
93	(1) 12 Kettlebell Clean and Press	Shoulders, Arms, Core	Clean kettlebell to shoulder, press overhead. Alternate arms. Complete 12 reps each arm.
	(2) 20 Air Squats	Legs, Glutes, Core	Stand, bend knees to lower body. Repeat for 20 reps.
	(3) 15 Kettlebell Bent Over Rows	Back, Shoulders, Arms	Hinge forward, row kettlebell to hip. Repeat for 15 reps each side.
	(4) 500-meter run	Legs, Cardio, Core	Run 500 meters at a steady pace.
	Repeat 5 times:		
94	(1) 40 seconds Kettlebell Snatch	Shoulders, Back, Core	Lift kettlebell overhead in one motion, lock arm. Alternate arms. Repeat for 40 seconds.
	(2) 20 seconds Rest		Rest for 20 seconds.
	(3) 40 seconds Burpees	Full Body, Core, Legs	Jump, squat down, kick back into push-up, return up. Repeat for 40 seconds.
	(4) 20 seconds Rest		Rest for 20 seconds.
	4 Rounds for time:		
95	(1) 20 Kettlebell Swings	Lower Body, Core, Shoulders	Swing kettlebell between legs, thrust hips forward. Repeat for 20 reps.
	(2) 20 Lunges	Legs, Glutes, Core	Step forward, lower hips to drop knee to ground. Repeat for 20 reps.
	(3) 15 Kettlebell Shoulder Press	Shoulders, Arms, Core	Press kettlebell overhead from shoulder level. Repeat for 15 reps each side.
	(4) 300-meter run	Legs, Cardio, Core	Run 300 meters at a steady pace.

Workout No.	Workout (Kettlebell & Body-Weight Workouts)	Main Muscle Groups	Instructions
96	**Repeat 5 times:**		
	(1) 45 seconds Kettlebell Around the Body	Core, Shoulders, Arms	Pass kettlebell around body, maintain core control. Repeat for 45 seconds.
	(2) 15 seconds Rest		Rest for 15 seconds.
	(3) 45 seconds Jumping Jacks	Cardio, Legs, Core	Jump to spread legs and clap hands overhead. Repeat for 45 seconds.
	(4) 15 seconds Rest		Rest for 15 seconds.
97	**3 Rounds for time:**		
	(1) 10 Kettlebell Snatches	Shoulders, Back, Core	Lift kettlebell overhead in one motion, lock arm. Alternate arms. Complete 10 reps each arm.
	(2) 20 Push-Ups	Chest, Triceps, Core	Lower body to ground, push up with arms. Repeat for 20 reps.
	(3) 15 Kettlebell Deadlifts	Lower Back, Hamstrings, Glutes	Lift kettlebell from ground, keep back straight. Repeat for 15 reps.
	(4) 300-meter run	Legs, Cardio, Core	Run 300 meters at a steady pace.
98	**Repeat 8 times:**		
	(1) 20 seconds Kettlebell Jump Swing	Legs, Core, Shoulders	Explosive swing with a jump at top of motion. Repeat for 20 seconds.
	(2) 10 seconds Rest		Rest for 10 seconds.
	(3) 20 seconds High Knees	Legs, Cardio, Core	Run in place lifting knees high. Repeat for 20 seconds.
	(4) 10 seconds Rest		Rest for 10 seconds.
99	**4 Rounds for time:**		
	(1) 15 Kettlebell Clean	Shoulders, Back, Core	Lift kettlebell to shoulder, flip grip at top. Repeat for 15 reps.
	(2) 20 V-Ups	Abs, Core, Hip Flexors	Lie back, lift legs and torso simultaneously. Repeat for 20 reps.
	(3) 20 Kettlebell Goblet Squats	Legs, Glutes, Core	Squat holding kettlebell close to chest. Repeat for 20 reps.
	(4) 250-meter run	Legs, Cardio, Core	Run 250 meters at a steady pace.
100	**Repeat 4 times with 1-minute rest between rounds:**		
	(1) 30 seconds Kettlebell Swing	Lower Body, Core, Shoulders	Swing kettlebell between legs, thrust hips forward, raise kettlebell to shoulder height. Repeat for 30 seconds.
	(2) 30 seconds Push-Ups	Chest, Triceps, Core	Lower body to ground, push up with arms. Repeat for 30 seconds.
	(3) 30 seconds Kettlebell Goblet Squats	Legs, Glutes, Core	Squat holding kettlebell close to chest. Repeat for 30 seconds.
	(4) 30 seconds Mountain Climbers	Cardio, Core, Legs	Run in place in plank position, drive knees to chest. Repeat for 30 seconds.

Workout No.	Workout (Kettlebell & Body-Weight Workouts)	Main Muscle Groups	Instructions
	4 Rounds for time:		
101	(1) 15 Kettlebell Deadlifts	Lower Back, Hamstrings, Glutes	Lift kettlebell from ground, keep back straight. Repeat for 15 reps.
	(2) 20 Push-Ups	Chest, Triceps, Core	Lower body to ground, push up with arms. Repeat for 20 reps.
	(3) 25 Kettlebell Goblet Squats	Legs, Glutes, Core	Squat holding kettlebell close to chest. Repeat for 25 reps.
	(4) 400-meter run	Legs, Cardio, Core	Run 400 meters at a steady pace.
	Repeat 4 times with 1-minute rest between rounds:		
102	(1) 30 seconds Kettlebell Swing	Lower Body, Core, Shoulders	Swing kettlebell between legs, thrust hips forward, raise kettlebell to shoulder height. Repeat for 30 seconds.
	(2) 30 seconds Mountain Climbers	Cardio, Core, Legs	Run in place in plank position, drive knees to chest. Repeat for 30 seconds.
	(3) 30 seconds Kettlebell Thrusters	Shoulders, Legs, Core	Squat to overhead press in one fluid motion. Repeat for 30 seconds.
	(4) 30 seconds Jumping Jacks	Cardio, Legs, Core	Jump to spread legs and clap hands overhead. Repeat for 30 seconds.
	3 Rounds for time:		
103	(1) 12 Kettlebell Clean and Press	Shoulders, Arms, Core	Clean kettlebell to shoulder, press overhead. Alternate arms. Complete 12 reps each arm.
	(2) 20 Air Squats	Legs, Glutes, Core	Stand, bend knees to lower body. Repeat for 20 reps.
	(3) 15 Kettlebell Bent Over Rows	Back, Shoulders, Arms	Hinge forward, row kettlebell to hip. Repeat for 15 reps each side.
	(4) 500-meter run	Legs, Cardio, Core	Run 500 meters at a steady pace.
	Repeat 5 times:		
104	(1) 40 seconds Kettlebell Snatch	Shoulders, Back, Core	Lift kettlebell overhead in one motion, lock arm. Alternate arms. Repeat for 40 seconds.
	(2) 20 seconds Rest		Rest for 20 seconds.
	(3) 40 seconds Burpees	Full Body, Core, Legs	Jump, squat down, kick back into push-up, return up. Repeat for 40 seconds.
	(4) 20 seconds Rest		Rest for 20 seconds.
	4 Rounds for time:		
105	(1) 20 Kettlebell Swings	Lower Body, Core, Shoulders	Swing kettlebell between legs, thrust hips forward. Repeat for 20 reps.
	(2) 20 Lunges	Legs, Glutes, Core	Step forward, lower hips to drop knee to ground. Repeat for 20 reps.
	(3) 15 Kettlebell Shoulder Press	Shoulders, Arms, Core	Press kettlebell overhead from shoulder level. Repeat for 15 reps each side.
	(4) 300-meter run	Legs, Cardio, Core	Run 300 meters at a steady pace.

Workout No.	Workout (Kettlebell & Body-Weight Workouts)	Main Muscle Groups	Instructions
106	**Repeat 5 times:**		
	(1) 45 seconds Kettlebell Around the Body	Core, Shoulders, Arms	Pass kettlebell around body, maintain core control. Repeat for 45 seconds.
	(2) 15 seconds Rest		Rest for 15 seconds.
	(3) 45 seconds Jumping Jacks	Cardio, Legs, Core	Jump to spread legs and clap hands overhead. Repeat for 45 seconds.
	(4) 15 seconds Rest		Rest for 15 seconds.
107	**3 Rounds for time:**		
	(1) 10 Kettlebell Snatches	Shoulders, Back, Core	Lift kettlebell overhead in one motion, lock arm. Alternate arms. Complete 10 reps each arm.
	(2) 20 Push-Ups	Chest, Triceps, Core	Lower body to ground, push up with arms. Repeat for 20 reps.
	(3) 15 Kettlebell Deadlifts	Lower Back, Hamstrings, Glutes	Lift kettlebell from ground, keep back straight. Repeat for 15 reps.
	(4) 300-meter run	Legs, Cardio, Core	Run 300 meters at a steady pace.
108	**Repeat 8 times:**		
	(1) 20 seconds Kettlebell Jump Swing	Legs, Core, Shoulders	Explosive swing with a jump at top of motion. Repeat for 20 seconds.
	(2) 10 seconds Rest		Rest for 10 seconds.
	(3) 20 seconds High Knees	Legs, Cardio, Core	Run in place lifting knees high. Repeat for 20 seconds.
	(4) 10 seconds Rest		Rest for 10 seconds.
109	**4 Rounds for time:**		
	(1) 15 Kettlebell Clean	Shoulders, Back, Core	Lift kettlebell to shoulder, flip grip at top. Repeat for 15 reps.
	(2) 20 V-Ups	Abs, Core, Hip Flexors	Lie back, lift legs and torso simultaneously. Repeat for 20 reps.
	(3) 20 Kettlebell Goblet Squats	Legs, Glutes, Core	Squat holding kettlebell close to chest. Repeat for 20 reps.
	(4) 250-meter run	Legs, Cardio, Core	Run 250 meters at a steady pace.
110	**Repeat 4 times with 1-minute rest between rounds:**		
	(1) 30 seconds Kettlebell Swing	Lower Body, Core, Shoulders	Swing kettlebell between legs, thrust hips forward, raise kettlebell to shoulder height. Repeat for 30 seconds.
	(2) 30 seconds Push-Ups	Chest, Triceps, Core	Lower body to ground, push up with arms. Repeat for 30 seconds.
	(3) 30 seconds Kettlebell Goblet Squats	Legs, Glutes, Core	Squat holding kettlebell close to chest. Repeat for 30 seconds.
	(4) 30 seconds Mountain Climbers	Cardio, Core, Legs	Run in place in plank position, drive knees to chest. Repeat for 30 seconds.

Workout No.	Workout (Kettlebell & Body-Weight Workouts)	Main Muscle Groups	Instructions
	4 Rounds for time:		
111	(1) 15 Kettlebell Swings	Lower Body, Core, Shoulders	Swing kettlebell between legs, thrust hips forward. Repeat for 15 reps.
	(2) 20 Air Squats	Legs, Glutes, Core	Stand, bend knees to lower body. Repeat for 20 reps.
	(3) 12 Kettlebell Clean and Press	Shoulders, Arms, Core	Clean kettlebell to shoulder, press overhead. Repeat for 12 reps each arm.
	(4) 400-meter run	Legs, Cardio, Core	Run 400 meters at a steady pace.
	Repeat 4 times with 1-minute rest between rounds:		
112	(1) 30 seconds Kettlebell Snatch	Shoulders, Back, Core	Lift kettlebell overhead in one motion. Alternate arms. Repeat for 30 seconds.
	(2) 30 seconds Mountain Climbers	Cardio, Core, Legs	Run in place in plank position, drive knees to chest. Repeat for 30 seconds.
	(3) 30 seconds Kettlebell Thrusters	Shoulders, Legs, Core	Squat to overhead press in one fluid motion. Repeat for 30 seconds.
	(4) 30 seconds Jumping Jacks	Cardio, Legs, Core	Jump to spread legs and clap hands overhead. Repeat for 30 seconds.
	3 Rounds for time:		
113	(1) 12 Kettlebell Deadlifts	Lower Back, Hamstrings, Glutes	Lift kettlebell from ground, keep back straight. Repeat for 12 reps.
	(2) 20 Push-Ups	Chest, Triceps, Core	Lower body to ground, push up with arms. Repeat for 20 reps.
	(3) 15 Kettlebell Bent Over Rows	Back, Shoulders, Arms	Hinge forward, row kettlebell to hip. Repeat for 15 reps each side.
	(4) 500-meter run	Legs, Cardio, Core	Run 500 meters at a steady pace.
	Repeat 5 times:		
114	(1) 40 seconds Kettlebell Around the Body	Core, Shoulders, Arms	Pass kettlebell around body, maintain core control. Repeat for 40 seconds.
	(2) 20 seconds Rest		Rest for 20 seconds.
	(3) 40 seconds Burpees	Full Body, Core, Legs	Jump, squat down, kick back into push-up, return up. Repeat for 40 seconds.
	(4) 20 seconds Rest		Rest for 20 seconds.
	4 Rounds for time:		
115	(1) 20 Kettlebell Snatches	Shoulders, Back, Core	Lift kettlebell overhead in one motion. Alternate arms. Repeat for 20 reps each arm.
	(2) 20 Lunges	Legs, Glutes, Core	Step forward, lower hips to drop knee to ground. Repeat for 20 reps.
	(3) 20 Kettlebell Goblet Squats	Legs, Glutes, Core	Squat holding kettlebell close to chest. Repeat for 20 reps.
	(4) 300-meter run	Legs, Cardio, Core	Run 300 meters at a steady pace.

Workout No.	Workout (Kettlebell & Body-Weight Workouts)	Main Muscle Groups	Instructions
116	**Repeat 5 times:**		
	(1) 45 seconds Kettlebell Jump Swing	Legs, Core, Shoulders	Explosive swing with a jump at top of motion. Repeat for 45 seconds.
	(2) 15 seconds Rest		Rest for 15 seconds.
	(3) 45 seconds Jumping Jacks	Cardio, Legs, Core	Jump to spread legs and clap hands overhead. Repeat for 45 seconds.
	(4) 15 seconds Rest		Rest for 15 seconds.
117	**3 Rounds for time:**		
	(1) 10 Kettlebell Clean and Press	Shoulders, Arms, Core	Clean kettlebell to shoulder, press overhead. Repeat for 10 reps each arm.
	(2) 20 Push-Ups	Chest, Triceps, Core	Lower body to ground, push up with arms. Repeat for 20 reps.
	(3) 15 Kettlebell Deadlifts	Lower Back, Hamstrings, Glutes	Lift kettlebell from ground, keep back straight. Repeat for 15 reps.
	(4) 300-meter run	Legs, Cardio, Core	Run 300 meters at a steady pace.
118	**Repeat 8 times:**		
	(1) 20 seconds Kettlebell Atlas Swing	Shoulders, Back, Core	Swing kettlebell up, catch at chest level. Repeat for 20 seconds.
	(2) 10 seconds Rest		Rest for 10 seconds.
	(3) 20 seconds High Knees	Legs, Cardio, Core	Run in place lifting knees high. Repeat for 20 seconds.
	(4) 10 seconds Rest		Rest for 10 seconds.
119	**4 Rounds for time:**		
	(1) 15 Kettlebell Clean	Shoulders, Back, Core	Lift kettlebell to shoulder, flip grip at top. Repeat for 15 reps.
	(2) 20 V-Ups	Abs, Core, Hip Flexors	Lie back, lift legs and torso simultaneously. Repeat for 20 reps.
	(3) 20 Kettlebell Goblet Squats	Legs, Glutes, Core	Squat holding kettlebell close to chest. Repeat for 20 reps.
	(4) 250-meter run	Legs, Cardio, Core	Run 250 meters at a steady pace.
120	**Repeat 4 times with 1-minute rest between rounds:**		
	(1) 30 seconds Kettlebell Swing	Lower Body, Core, Shoulders	Swing kettlebell between legs, thrust hips forward, raise kettlebell to shoulder height. Repeat for 30 seconds.
	(2) 30 seconds Push-Ups	Chest, Triceps, Core	Lower body to ground, push up with arms. Repeat for 30 seconds.
	(3) 30 seconds Kettlebell Goblet Squats	Legs, Glutes, Core	Squat holding kettlebell close to chest. Repeat for 30 seconds.
	(4) 30 seconds Mountain Climbers	Cardio, Core, Legs	Run in place in plank position, drive knees to chest. Repeat for 30 seconds.

Workout No.	Workout (Kettlebell & Body-Weight Workouts)	Main Muscle Groups	Instructions
	4 Rounds for time:		
	(1) 15 Kettlebell Swings	Lower Body, Core, Shoulders	Swing kettlebell between legs, thrust hips forward. Repeat for 15 reps.
121	(2) 20 Air Squats	Legs, Glutes, Core	Stand, bend knees to lower body. Repeat for 20 reps.
	(3) 12 Kettlebell Clean and Press	Shoulders, Arms, Core	Clean kettlebell to shoulder, press overhead. Repeat for 12 reps each arm.
	(4) 400-meter run	Legs, Cardio, Core	Run 400 meters at a steady pace.
	Repeat 4 times with 1-minute rest between rounds:		
	(1) 30 seconds Kettlebell Snatch	Shoulders, Back, Core	Lift kettlebell overhead in one motion. Alternate arms. Repeat for 30 seconds.
122	(2) 30 seconds Mountain Climbers	Cardio, Core, Legs	Run in place in plank position, drive knees to chest. Repeat for 30 seconds.
	(3) 30 seconds Kettlebell Thrusters	Shoulders, Legs, Core	Squat to overhead press in one fluid motion. Repeat for 30 seconds.
	(4) 30 seconds Jumping Jacks	Cardio, Legs, Core	Jump to spread legs and clap hands overhead. Repeat for 30 seconds.
	3 Rounds for time:		
	(1) 12 Kettlebell Deadlifts	Lower Back, Hamstrings, Glutes	Lift kettlebell from ground, keep back straight. Repeat for 12 reps.
123	(2) 20 Push-Ups	Chest, Triceps, Core	Lower body to ground, push up with arms. Repeat for 20 reps.
	(3) 15 Kettlebell Bent Over Rows	Back, Shoulders, Arms	Hinge forward, row kettlebell to hip. Repeat for 15 reps each side.
	(4) 500-meter run	Legs, Cardio, Core	Run 500 meters at a steady pace.
	Repeat 5 times:		
	(1) 40 seconds Kettlebell Around the Body	Core, Shoulders, Arms	Pass kettlebell around body, maintain core control. Repeat for 40 seconds.
124	(2) 20 seconds Rest		Rest for 20 seconds.
	(3) 40 seconds Burpees	Full Body, Core, Legs	Jump, squat down, kick back into push-up, return up. Repeat for 40 seconds.
	(4) 20 seconds Rest		Rest for 20 seconds.
	4 Rounds for time:		
	(1) 20 Kettlebell Snatches	Shoulders, Back, Core	Lift kettlebell overhead in one motion. Alternate arms. Repeat for 20 reps each arm.
125	(2) 20 Lunges	Legs, Glutes, Core	Step forward, lower hips to drop knee to ground. Repeat for 20 reps.
	(3) 20 Kettlebell Goblet Squats	Legs, Glutes, Core	Squat holding kettlebell close to chest. Repeat for 20 reps.
	(4) 300-meter run	Legs, Cardio, Core	Run 300 meters at a steady pace.

Workout No.	Workout (Kettlebell & Body-Weight Workouts)	Main Muscle Groups	Instructions
126	**Repeat 5 times:**		
	(1) 45 seconds Kettlebell Jump Swing	Legs, Core, Shoulders	Explosive swing with a jump at top of motion. Repeat for 45 seconds.
	(2) 15 seconds Rest		Rest for 15 seconds.
	(3) 45 seconds Jumping Jacks	Cardio, Legs, Core	Jump to spread legs and clap hands overhead. Repeat for 45 seconds.
	(4) 15 seconds Rest		Rest for 15 seconds.
127	**3 Rounds for time:**		
	(1) 10 Kettlebell Clean and Press	Shoulders, Arms, Core	Clean kettlebell to shoulder, press overhead. Repeat for 10 reps each arm.
	(2) 20 Push-Ups	Chest, Triceps, Core	Lower body to ground, push up with arms. Repeat for 20 reps.
	(3) 15 Kettlebell Deadlifts	Lower Back, Hamstrings, Glutes	Lift kettlebell from ground, keep back straight. Repeat for 15 reps.
	(4) 300-meter run	Legs, Cardio, Core	Run 300 meters at a steady pace.
128	**Repeat 8 times:**		
	(1) 20 seconds Kettlebell Atlas Swing	Shoulders, Back, Core	Swing kettlebell up, catch at chest level. Repeat for 20 seconds.
	(2) 10 seconds Rest		Rest for 10 seconds.
	(3) 20 seconds High Knees	Legs, Cardio, Core	Run in place lifting knees high. Repeat for 20 seconds.
	(4) 10 seconds Rest		Rest for 10 seconds.
129	**4 Rounds for time:**		
	(1) 15 Kettlebell Clean	Shoulders, Back, Core	Lift kettlebell to shoulder, flip grip at top. Repeat for 15 reps.
	(2) 20 V-Ups	Abs, Core, Hip Flexors	Lie back, lift legs and torso simultaneously. Repeat for 20 reps.
	(3) 20 Kettlebell Goblet Squats	Legs, Glutes, Core	Squat holding kettlebell close to chest. Repeat for 20 reps.
	(4) 250-meter run	Legs, Cardio, Core	Run 250 meters at a steady pace.
130	**Repeat 4 times with 1-minute rest between rounds:**		
	(1) 30 seconds Kettlebell Swing	Lower Body, Core, Shoulders	Swing kettlebell between legs, thrust hips forward, raise kettlebell to shoulder height. Repeat for 30 seconds.
	(2) 30 seconds Push-Ups	Chest, Triceps, Core	Lower body to ground, push up with arms. Repeat for 30 seconds.
	(3) 30 seconds Kettlebell Goblet Squats	Legs, Glutes, Core	Squat holding kettlebell close to chest. Repeat for 30 seconds.
	(4) 30 seconds Mountain Climbers	Cardio, Core, Legs	Run in place in plank position, drive knees to chest. Repeat for 30 seconds.

Workout No.	Workout (Kettlebell & Body-Weight Workouts)	Main Muscle Groups	Instructions
131	**4 Rounds for time:**		
	(1) 15 Kettlebell Swings	Lower Body, Core, Shoulders	Swing kettlebell between legs, thrust hips forward. Repeat for 15 reps.
	(2) 20 Air Squats	Legs, Glutes, Core	Stand, bend knees to lower body. Repeat for 20 reps.
	(3) 12 Kettlebell Clean and Press	Shoulders, Arms, Core	Clean kettlebell to shoulder, press overhead. Repeat for 12 reps each arm.
	(4) 400-meter run	Legs, Cardio, Core	Run 400 meters at a steady pace.
132	**Repeat 4 times with 1-minute rest between rounds:**		
	(1) 30 seconds Kettlebell Snatch	Shoulders, Back, Core	Lift kettlebell overhead in one motion. Alternate arms. Repeat for 30 seconds.
	(2) 30 seconds Mountain Climbers	Cardio, Core, Legs	Run in place in plank position, drive knees to chest. Repeat for 30 seconds.
	(3) 30 seconds Kettlebell Thrusters	Shoulders, Legs, Core	Squat to overhead press in one fluid motion. Repeat for 30 seconds.
	(4) 30 seconds Jumping Jacks	Cardio, Legs, Core	Jump to spread legs and clap hands overhead. Repeat for 30 seconds.
133	**3 Rounds for time:**		
	(1) 12 Kettlebell Deadlifts	Lower Back, Hamstrings, Glutes	Lift kettlebell from ground, keep back straight. Repeat for 12 reps.
	(2) 20 Push-Ups	Chest, Triceps, Core	Lower body to ground, push up with arms. Repeat for 20 reps.
	(3) 15 Kettlebell Bent Over Rows	Back, Shoulders, Arms	Hinge forward, row kettlebell to hip. Repeat for 15 reps each side.
	(4) 500-meter run	Legs, Cardio, Core	Run 500 meters at a steady pace.
134	**Repeat 5 times:**		
	(1) 40 seconds Kettlebell Around the Body	Core, Shoulders, Arms	Pass kettlebell around body, maintain core control. Repeat for 40 seconds.
	(2) 20 seconds Rest		Rest for 20 seconds.
	(3) 40 seconds Burpees	Full Body, Core, Legs	Jump, squat down, kick back into push-up, return up. Repeat for 40 seconds.
	(4) 20 seconds Rest		Rest for 20 seconds.
135	**4 Rounds for time:**		
	(1) 20 Kettlebell Snatches	Shoulders, Back, Core	Lift kettlebell overhead in one motion. Alternate arms. Repeat for 20 reps each arm.
	(2) 20 Lunges	Legs, Glutes, Core	Step forward, lower hips to drop knee to ground. Repeat for 20 reps.
	(3) 20 Kettlebell Goblet Squats	Legs, Glutes, Core	Squat holding kettlebell close to chest. Repeat for 20 reps.
	(4) 300-meter run	Legs, Cardio, Core	Run 300 meters at a steady pace.

Workout No.	Workout (Kettlebell & Body-Weight Workouts)	Main Muscle Groups	Instructions
136	**Repeat 5 times:**		
	(1) 45 seconds Kettlebell Jump Swing	Legs, Core, Shoulders	Explosive swing with a jump at top of motion. Repeat for 45 seconds.
	(2) 15 seconds Rest		Rest for 15 seconds.
	(3) 45 seconds Jumping Jacks	Cardio, Legs, Core	Jump to spread legs and clap hands overhead. Repeat for 45 seconds.
	(4) 15 seconds Rest		Rest for 15 seconds.
137	**3 Rounds for time:**		
	(1) 10 Kettlebell Clean and Press	Shoulders, Arms, Core	Clean kettlebell to shoulder, press overhead. Repeat for 10 reps each arm.
	(2) 20 Push-Ups	Chest, Triceps, Core	Lower body to ground, push up with arms. Repeat for 20 reps.
	(3) 15 Kettlebell Deadlifts	Lower Back, Hamstrings, Glutes	Lift kettlebell from ground, keep back straight. Repeat for 15 reps.
	(4) 300-meter run	Legs, Cardio, Core	Run 300 meters at a steady pace.
138	**Repeat 8 times:**		
	(1) 20 seconds Kettlebell Atlas Swing	Shoulders, Back, Core	Swing kettlebell up, catch at chest level. Repeat for 20 seconds.
	(2) 10 seconds Rest		Rest for 10 seconds.
	(3) 20 seconds High Knees	Legs, Cardio, Core	Run in place lifting knees high. Repeat for 20 seconds.
	(4) 10 seconds Rest		Rest for 10 seconds.
139	**4 Rounds for time:**		
	(1) 15 Kettlebell Clean	Shoulders, Back, Core	Lift kettlebell to shoulder, flip grip at top. Repeat for 15 reps.
	(2) 20 V-Ups	Abs, Core, Hip Flexors	Lie back, lift legs and torso simultaneously. Repeat for 20 reps.
	(3) 20 Kettlebell Goblet Squats	Legs, Glutes, Core	Squat holding kettlebell close to chest. Repeat for 20 reps.
	(4) 250-meter run	Legs, Cardio, Core	Run 250 meters at a steady pace.
140	**Repeat 4 times with 1-minute rest between rounds:**		
	(1) 30 seconds Kettlebell Swing	Lower Body, Core, Shoulders	Swing kettlebell between legs, thrust hips forward, raise kettlebell to shoulder height. Repeat for 30 seconds.
	(2) 30 seconds Push-Ups	Chest, Triceps, Core	Lower body to ground, push up with arms. Repeat for 30 seconds.
	(3) 30 seconds Kettlebell Goblet Squats	Legs, Glutes, Core	Squat holding kettlebell close to chest. Repeat for 30 seconds.
	(4) 30 seconds Mountain Climbers	Cardio, Core, Legs	Run in place in plank position, drive knees to chest. Repeat for 30 seconds.

Workout No.	Workout (Kettlebell & Body-Weight Workouts)	Main Muscle Groups	Instructions
	4 Rounds for time:		
141	(1) 15 Kettlebell Swings	Lower Body, Core, Shoulders	Swing kettlebell between legs, thrust hips forward. Repeat for 15 reps.
	(2) 20 Air Squats	Legs, Glutes, Core	Stand, bend knees to lower body. Repeat for 20 reps.
	(3) 12 Kettlebell Clean and Press	Shoulders, Arms, Core	Clean kettlebell to shoulder, press overhead. Repeat for 12 reps each arm.
	(4) 400-meter run	Legs, Cardio, Core	Run 400 meters at a steady pace.
	Repeat 4 times with 1-minute rest between rounds:		
142	(1) 30 seconds Kettlebell Snatch	Shoulders, Back, Core	Lift kettlebell overhead in one motion. Alternate arms. Repeat for 30 seconds.
	(2) 30 seconds Mountain Climbers	Cardio, Core, Legs	Run in place in plank position, drive knees to chest. Repeat for 30 seconds.
	(3) 30 seconds Kettlebell Thrusters	Shoulders, Legs, Core	Squat to overhead press in one fluid motion. Repeat for 30 seconds.
	(4) 30 seconds Jumping Jacks	Cardio, Legs, Core	Jump to spread legs and clap hands overhead. Repeat for 30 seconds.
	3 Rounds for time:		
143	(1) 12 Kettlebell Deadlifts	Lower Back, Hamstrings, Glutes	Lift kettlebell from ground, keep back straight. Repeat for 12 reps.
	(2) 20 Push-Ups	Chest, Triceps, Core	Lower body to ground, push up with arms. Repeat for 20 reps.
	(3) 15 Kettlebell Bent Over Rows	Back, Shoulders, Arms	Hinge forward, row kettlebell to hip. Repeat for 15 reps each side.
	(4) 500-meter run	Legs, Cardio, Core	Run 500 meters at a steady pace.
	Repeat 5 times:		
144	(1) 40 seconds Kettlebell Around the Body	Core, Shoulders, Arms	Pass kettlebell around body, maintain core control. Repeat for 40 seconds.
	(2) 20 seconds Rest		Rest for 20 seconds.
	(3) 40 seconds Burpees	Full Body, Core, Legs	Jump, squat down, kick back into push-up, return up. Repeat for 40 seconds.
	(4) 20 seconds Rest		Rest for 20 seconds.
	4 Rounds for time:		
145	(1) 20 Kettlebell Snatches	Shoulders, Back, Core	Lift kettlebell overhead in one motion. Alternate arms. Repeat for 20 reps each arm.
	(2) 20 Lunges	Legs, Glutes, Core	Step forward, lower hips to drop knee to ground. Repeat for 20 reps.
	(3) 20 Kettlebell Goblet Squats	Legs, Glutes, Core	Squat holding kettlebell close to chest. Repeat for 20 reps.
	(4) 300-meter run	Legs, Cardio, Core	Run 300 meters at a steady pace.

Workout No.	Workout (Kettlebell & Body-Weight Workouts)	Main Muscle Groups	Instructions
146	**Repeat 5 times:**		
	45 seconds Kettlebell Jump Swing	Legs, Core, Shoulders	Explosive swing with a jump at top of motion. Repeat for 45 seconds.
	15 seconds Rest		Rest for 15 seconds.
	45 seconds Jumping Jacks	Cardio, Legs, Core	Jump to spread legs and clap hands overhead. Repeat for 45 seconds.
	15 seconds Rest		Rest for 15 seconds.
147	**3 Rounds for time:**		
	(1) 10 Kettlebell Clean and Press	Shoulders, Arms, Core	Clean kettlebell to shoulder, press overhead. Repeat for 10 reps each arm.
	(2) 20 Push-Ups	Chest, Triceps, Core	Lower body to ground, push up with arms. Repeat for 20 reps.
	(3) 15 Kettlebell Deadlifts	Lower Back, Hamstrings, Glutes	Lift kettlebell from ground, keep back straight. Repeat for 15 reps.
	(4) 300-meter run	Legs, Cardio, Core	Run 300 meters at a steady pace.
148	**Repeat 8 times:**		
	(1) 20 seconds Kettlebell Atlas Swing	Shoulders, Back, Core	Swing kettlebell up, catch at chest level. Repeat for 20 seconds.
	(2) 10 seconds Rest		Rest for 10 seconds.
	(3) 20 seconds High Knees	Legs, Cardio, Core	Run in place lifting knees high. Repeat for 20 seconds.
	(4) 10 seconds Rest		Rest for 10 seconds.
149	**4 Rounds for time:**		
	(1) 15 Kettlebell Clean	Shoulders, Back, Core	Lift kettlebell to shoulder, flip grip at top. Repeat for 15 reps.
	(2) 20 V-Ups	Abs, Core, Hip Flexors	Lie back, lift legs and torso simultaneously. Repeat for 20 reps.
	(3) 20 Kettlebell Goblet Squats	Legs, Glutes, Core	Squat holding kettlebell close to chest. Repeat for 20 reps.
	(4) 250-meter run	Legs, Cardio, Core	Run 250 meters at a steady pace.
150	**Repeat 4 times with 1-minute rest between rounds:**		
	(1) 30 seconds Kettlebell Swing	Lower Body, Core, Shoulders	Swing kettlebell between legs, thrust hips forward, raise kettlebell to shoulder height. Repeat for 30 seconds.
	(2) 30 seconds Push-Ups	Chest, Triceps, Core	Lower body to ground, push up with arms. Repeat for 30 seconds.
	(3) 30 seconds Kettlebell Goblet Squats	Legs, Glutes, Core	Squat holding kettlebell close to chest. Repeat for 30 seconds.
	(4) 30 seconds Mountain Climbers	Cardio, Core, Legs	Run in place in plank position, drive knees to chest. Repeat for 30 seconds.

Body-Weight Exercises Guide

Body-Weight Exercises

Alternate Arm/Leg Plank

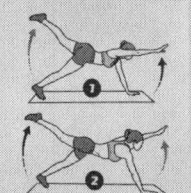

Plank, extend opposite arm and leg, hold.

1. Start in a plank position with hands directly under shoulders.
2. Simultaneously lift and extend your right arm and left leg.
3. Hold this position for a few seconds.
4. Return to the plank position.
5. Repeat with the left arm and right leg.

Army Crawl

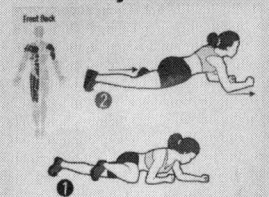

Crawl flat on stomach, using elbows and knees.

1. Lie flat on your stomach with elbows bent and hands directly in front of you.
2. Push with your toes and pull with your elbows to crawl forward.
3. Keep your body low and hips down.
4. Continue crawling for the desired distance or time.

Back Bridge

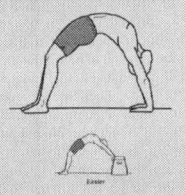

Plank, extend opposite arm and leg, hold.

1. Lie on your back with knees bent and feet flat on the floor.
2. Place your hands palms down by your sides.
3. Press through your feet and lift your hips up towards the ceiling.
4. Hold this position, squeezing your glutes and keeping your core tight.
5. Lower your hips back down to the starting position.

Bear Crawl

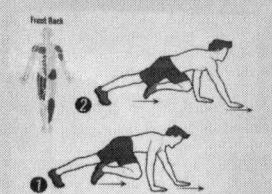

Crawl forward on all fours, hips down, move quickly.

1. Start on all fours with hands under shoulders and knees under hips.
2. Lift your knees slightly off the ground, keeping your back flat.
3. Move your right hand and left foot forward simultaneously.
4. Follow with your left hand and right foot, maintaining a low position.
5. Continue moving forward in this manner quickly.

Bicycle Crunches

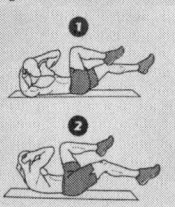

Lie down, alternate elbows to opposite knees cycling legs.

1. Lie on your back with hands behind your head and knees bent.
2. Lift your shoulders off the ground and bring your right elbow towards your left knee while extending the right leg.
3. Switch sides, bringing your left elbow towards your right knee while extending the left leg.
4. Continue alternating sides in a pedaling motion.

Bird Dog

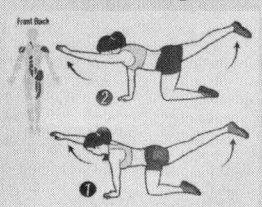

Extend opposite arm and leg, kneeling position.

1. Start on all fours with hands under shoulders and knees under hips.
2. Extend your right arm forward and your left leg backward simultaneously.
3. Hold for a few seconds, keeping your core engaged.
4. Return to the starting position.
5. Repeat with the left arm and right leg.

Bodyweight Row

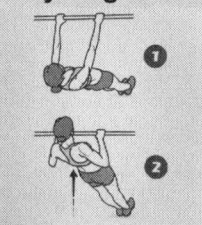

Pull body up towards a bar or table, lying underneath.

1. Position yourself under a bar or table, gripping it with both hands.
2. Keep your body straight and pull your chest up towards the bar.
3. Hold for a moment at the top of the movement.
4. Lower yourself back down to the starting position.
5. Repeat for the desired number of repetitions.

Burpee

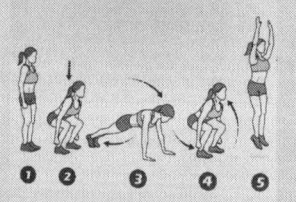

Jump, squat down, kick back into a push-up, return up.

1. Start standing with feet shoulder-width apart.
2. Drop into a squat position and place your hands on the ground.
3. Kick your feet back into a push-up position and lower your body to the ground.
4. Push back up to the push-up position and jump your feet back to your hands.
5. Explosively jump into the air, reaching your arms overhead.
6. Land softly and repeat.

Calf Raise

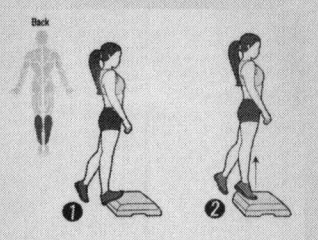

Raise heels off ground, balance on toes, lower slowly.

1. Stand with feet hip-width apart on a flat surface or step.
2. Lift your heels off the ground, balancing on the balls of your feet.
3. Hold the position for a second.
4. Slowly lower your heels back to the ground.
5. Repeat for the desired number of repetitions.

Calf Raises

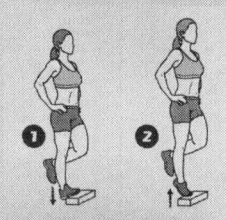

Lift heels off ground, balance on toes, lower slowly.

1. Stand with feet hip-width apart on a flat surface or step.
2. Lift your heels off the ground, balancing on the balls of your feet.
3. Hold the position for a second.
4. Slowly lower your heels back to the ground.
5. Repeat for the desired number of repetitions.

Cat/Camel

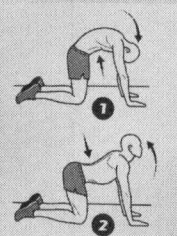

On hands and knees, arch back up and down.

1. Start on all fours with hands under shoulders and knees under hips.
2. Arch your back up towards the ceiling (Cat position).
3. Hold for a few seconds.
4. Lower your back down and lift your head and tailbone up (Camel position).
5. Alternate between the two positions, moving slowly and smoothly.

Crab Toe Touch

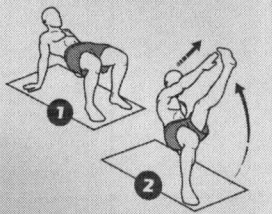

Crawl forward on all fours, hips down, move quickly.

1. Sit on the ground with knees bent, feet flat, and hands behind you.
2. Lift your hips off the ground into a crab position.
3. Reach your right hand to touch your left foot while lifting it.
4. Return to the starting position.
5. Repeat with the left hand and right foot, alternating sides.

Crab Walk

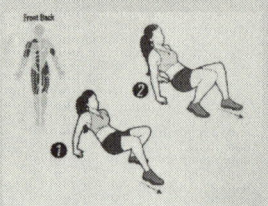

Walk backward on hands and feet, hips elevated.

1. Sit on the ground with knees bent, feet flat, and hands behind you.
2. Lift your hips off the ground into a crab position.
3. Walk backward using your hands and feet, keeping hips elevated.
4. Continue for the desired distance or time.

Crocodile Crawl

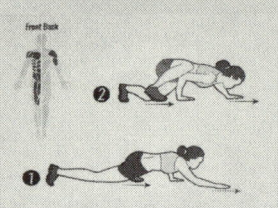

Crawl forward lying almost flat, use elbows and toes.

1. Start in a plank position with elbows bent and body low to the ground.
2. Move forward by simultaneously pulling with one arm and pushing with the opposite leg.
3. Keep your body as low and flat as possible.
4. Continue crawling forward for the desired distance or time.

Cross-Body Crunch

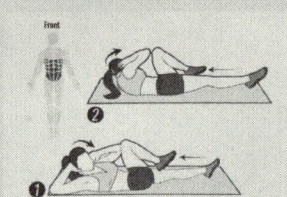

Touch opposite knee to elbow, lying down.

1. Lie on your back with knees bent and hands behind your head.
2. Lift your shoulders off the ground and bring your right elbow towards your left knee while extending the right leg.
3. Return to the starting position.
4. Repeat with the left elbow towards the right knee, alternating sides.

Crunch

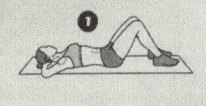

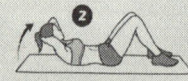

Lift shoulders off ground, contract abdominals.

1. Lie on your back with knees bent and feet flat on the ground.
2. Place your hands behind your head without pulling on your neck.
3. Lift your shoulders off the ground by contracting your abdominal muscles.
4. Hold for a second at the top.
5. Slowly lower back down to the starting position.

Dolphin Kick

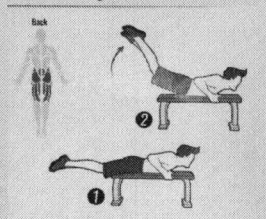

Lie face down, kick legs like a dolphin's tail.

1. Lie face down on a bench with your hips at the edge.
2. Hold onto the bench for support.
3. Lift your legs off the ground, keeping them straight.
4. Kick your legs up and down like a dolphin's tail.
5. Continue for the desired number of repetitions or time.

Donkey Kicks

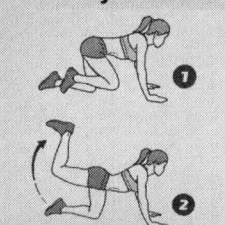

On hands and knees, kick one leg back and up.

1. Start on all fours with hands under shoulders and knees under hips.
2. Keep your right knee bent and lift your right leg up towards the ceiling.
3. Squeeze your glutes at the top.
4. Lower your leg back down without touching the ground.
5. Repeat on the other leg.

Fire Hydrant

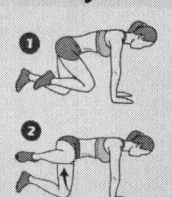

On hands and knees, lift leg to side, keep knee bent.

1. Start on all fours with hands under shoulders and knees under hips.
2. Keep your right knee bent and lift it out to the side.
3. Hold for a moment at the top.
4. Lower your knee back down without touching the ground.
5. Repeat on the other leg.

Flutter Kicks

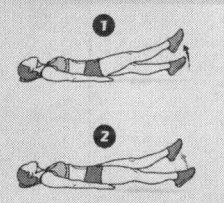

Lie on back, alternately kick legs in small, rapid motion.

1. Lie on your back with hands under your hips for support.
2. Lift both legs off the ground slightly.
3. Alternately kick your legs up and down in a small, rapid motion.
4. Keep your core engaged and back flat on the ground.
5. Continue for the desired time.

Glute Bridge

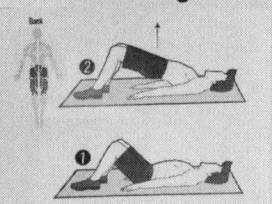

Lift hips while lying on back, feet flat on ground.

1. Lie on your back with knees bent and feet flat on the ground.
2. Place your arms by your sides with palms down.
3. Lift your hips towards the ceiling by squeezing your glutes.
4. Hold for a moment at the top.
5. Lower your hips back to the starting position.

Good Morning

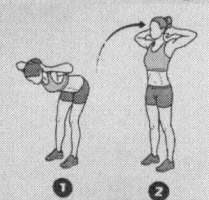

Hinge at hips with hands behind head, focus on hamstrings.

1. Stand with feet shoulder-width apart and hands behind your head.
2. Keep your back straight and hinge at the hips, bending forward.
3. Lower your torso until it's parallel to the ground.
4. Focus on feeling the stretch in your hamstrings.
5. Return to the starting position by engaging your glutes and hamstrings.

Hanging Knee Raise

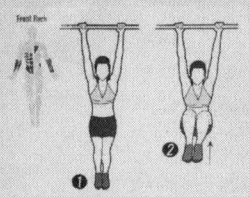

Hang from bar, raise knees towards chest.

1. Hang from a bar with arms extended and feet off the ground.
2. Keep your legs straight and together.
3. Lift your knees towards your chest by engaging your core.
4. Hold for a moment at the top.
5. Lower your legs back to the starting position.

High Knees

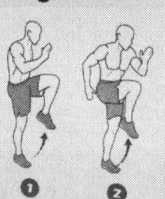

Run in place lifting knees high, maintain pace.

1. Stand with feet hip-width apart.
2. Run in place, lifting your knees as high as possible.
3. Pump your arms in coordination with your legs.
4. Maintain a quick pace and keep your core engaged.
5. Continue for the desired time.

Hip Raise

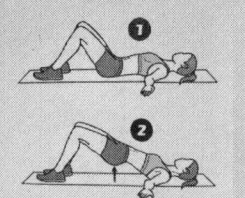

Lift hips while lying on back, feet flat on ground.

1. Lie on your back with knees bent and feet flat on the ground.
2. Place your arms by your sides with palms down.
3. Lift your hips towards the ceiling by squeezing your glutes.
4. Hold for a moment at the top.
5. Lower your hips back to the starting position.
6. Repeat for the desired number of repetitions.

Inchworm

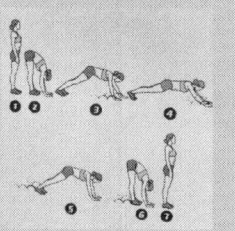

Walk hands forward from standing, hold plank, walk back.

1. Stand with feet hip-width apart.
2. Bend at the waist and place your hands on the ground.
3. Walk your hands forward until you are in a plank position.
4. Hold the plank for a few seconds.
5. Walk your hands back towards your feet and stand up.
6. Repeat for the desired number of repetitions.

Jumping Jacks

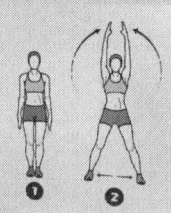

Jump to spread legs and clap hands overhead.

1. Stand with feet together and arms at your sides.
2. Jump to spread your legs while raising your arms overhead to clap.
3. Jump back to the starting position with feet together and arms at your sides.
4. Maintain a quick pace and keep your movements controlled.
5. Repeat for the desired number of repetitions or time.

Leg Pull-In

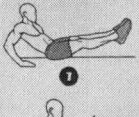

Sit, pull knees into chest, extend legs out.

1. Sit on the ground with legs extended and hands behind you for support.
2. Lean back slightly and lift your legs off the ground.
3. Pull your knees into your chest.
4. Extend your legs back out without touching the ground.
5. Repeat for the desired number of repetitions.

Lunge

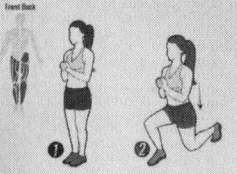

Step forward, lower hips to drop knee to ground.

1. Stand with feet hip-width apart.
2. Step forward with your right leg and lower your hips to drop your right knee towards the ground.
3. Ensure your right knee is directly above your ankle.
4. Push through your right heel to return to the starting position.
5. Repeat with the left leg, alternating sides.

Lying Leg Lift

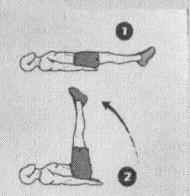

Raise legs vertically, lying flat on back.

1. Lie flat on your back with legs extended and arms by your sides.
2. Keep your legs straight and lift them towards the ceiling until they form a 90-degree angle with your torso.
3. Hold for a moment at the top.
4. Lower your legs back down without touching the ground.
5. Repeat for the desired number of repetitions.

Mountain Climber

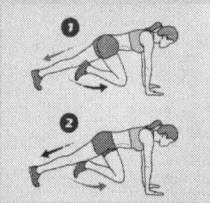

Run in place in plank position, drive knees to chest.

1. Start in a plank position with hands under shoulders and body in a straight line.
2. Bring your right knee towards your chest.
3. Quickly switch legs, bringing your left knee towards your chest while extending your right leg back.
4. Continue alternating legs in a running motion.
5. Maintain a quick pace and keep your core engaged.

Pike Push Up

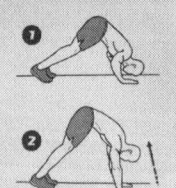

Push-up with hips high, resembles downward dog pose.

1. Start in a downward dog position with hips high and hands shoulder-width apart.
2. Lower your head towards the ground by bending your elbows.
3. Push through your hands to return to the starting position.
4. Keep your body in an inverted V shape throughout the movement.
5. Repeat for the desired number of repetitions.

Plank Rotation

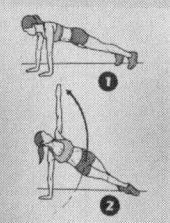

Rotate body in plank, extend arm upward, switch sides.

1. Stand with feet hip-width apart.
2. Step forward with your right leg and lower your hips to drop your right knee towards the ground.
3. Ensure your right knee is directly above your ankle.
4. Push through your right heel to return to the starting position.
5. Repeat with the left leg, alternating sides.

Pull Up

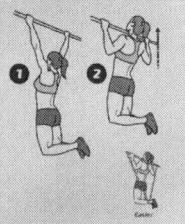

Pull body up on bar, chin above hands.

1. Hang from a pull-up bar with hands shoulder-width apart and palms facing away.
2. Engage your core and pull your body up until your chin is above the bar.
3. Hold for a moment at the top.
4. Lower yourself back down to the starting position with control.
5. Repeat for the desired number of repetitions.

Push Up

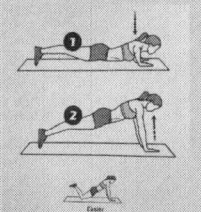

Lower body to ground, push up with arms.

1. Start in a plank position with hands slightly wider than shoulder-width apart.
2. Lower your body towards the ground by bending your elbows.
3. Keep your body in a straight line from head to heels.
4. Push through your hands to return to the starting position.
5. Repeat for the desired number of repetitions.

Push-Back

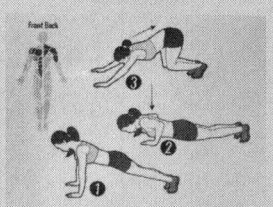

Push body back from push-up position to heels.

1. Start in a plank position with hands under shoulders.
2. Push your hips back towards your heels while keeping your arms extended.
3. Lower your chest towards the ground.
4. Return to the starting plank position.
5. Repeat for the desired number of repetitions.

Push-Up w/ Extension

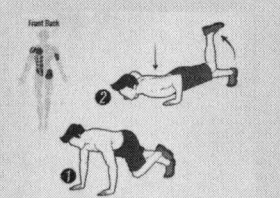

Perform push-up, extend one arm forward, alternate.

1. Start in a plank position with hands under shoulders.
2. Perform a push-up by lowering your body to the ground.
3. As you push back up, extend your right arm forward.
4. Return your hand to the ground.
5. Repeat with the left arm, alternating sides.

Reverse Crunch

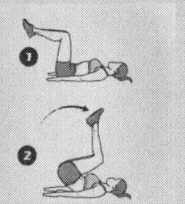

Lift hips off floor, knees towards chest.

1. Lie on your back with knees bent and feet flat on the ground.
2. Place your hands by your sides or under your hips for support.
3. Lift your hips off the ground and bring your knees towards your chest.
4. Hold for a moment at the top.
5. Lower your hips back to the starting position.
6. Repeat for the desired number of repetitions.

Reverse Plank

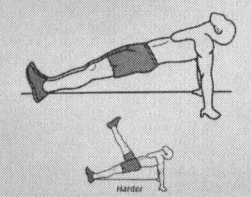

Sit, lift body with arms, legs straight, face up.

1. Sit on the ground with legs extended and hands behind you, fingers pointing forward.
2. Lift your hips off the ground by pressing through your hands and heels.
3. Keep your body in a straight line from head to heels.
4. Hold for the desired time.
5. Lower your hips back to the ground.

Russian Twist

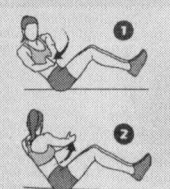

Twist torso holding weight, seated on ground.

1. Sit on the ground with knees bent and feet flat.
2. Lean back slightly and lift your feet off the ground, balancing on your sit bones.
3. Hold a weight with both hands and twist your torso to the right, bringing the weight beside your hip.
4. Twist to the left, bringing the weight to the other side.
5. Continue alternating sides for the desired number of repetitions.

Scissor Kick

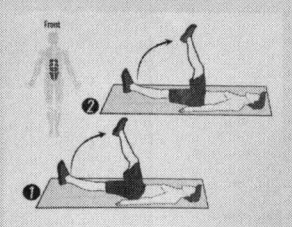

Alternately lift legs in lying position, engages core.

1. Lie flat on your back with hands under your hips for support.
2. Lift your legs slightly off the ground.
3. Alternately lift one leg higher while lowering the other leg, keeping both legs straight.
4. Continue the scissor motion, engaging your core throughout.
5. Repeat for the desired number of repetitions or time.

Side Crunches

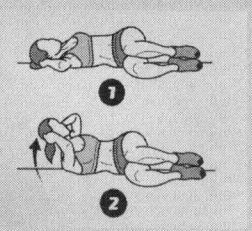

Lie on side, perform crunches towards elevated leg.

1. Lie on your side with legs bent and hands behind your head.
2. Lift your upper body towards your hips, crunching towards the elevated leg.
3. Squeeze your obliques at the top of the movement.
4. Lower back down to the starting position.
5. Repeat for the desired number of repetitions, then switch sides.

Side Lunge

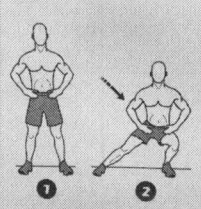

Step to side into lunge, keep other leg straight.

1. Stand with feet hip-width apart.
2. Step to the side with your right leg, lowering your hips into a lunge.
3. Keep your left leg straight and your chest up.
4. Push through your right foot to return to the starting position.
5. Repeat on the other side, alternating legs.

Side Plank

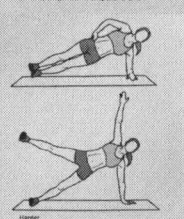

Support body on one arm, side facing ground.

1. Lie on your side with your elbow directly under your shoulder.
2. Lift your hips off the ground, forming a straight line from head to feet.
3. Hold this position, keeping your core engaged.
4. For added difficulty, extend your top arm towards the ceiling.
5. Repeat on the other side.

Side-to-Side Pull-Up

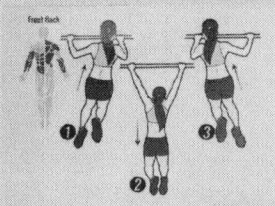

Pull up and move sideways along bar, alternate sides.

1. Hang from a pull-up bar with hands shoulder-width apart.
2. Pull your body up towards the bar, moving to the right side.
3. Lower yourself back down and pull up again, moving to the left side.
4. Continue alternating sides.
5. Repeat for the desired number of repetitions.

Side-to-Side Push-Up

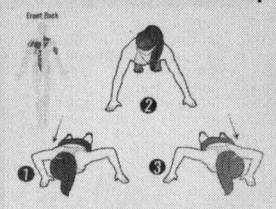

Shift side-to-side during push-ups, engages core.

1. Start in a plank position with hands slightly wider than shoulder-width apart.
2. Lower your body towards the ground, shifting your weight to the right.
3. Push back up and shift your weight to the left.
4. Continue alternating sides with each push-up.
5. Repeat for the desired number of repetitions.

Single Leg Dead Lift

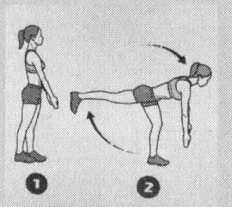

Balance on one leg, hinge forward, extend free leg back.

1. Stand on your right leg with a slight bend in the knee.
2. Hinge at the hips, extending your left leg back and lowering your torso towards the ground.
3. Keep your back straight and core engaged.
4. Return to the starting position by squeezing your glutes.
5. Repeat on the other leg, alternating sides.

Single Leg Split Squat

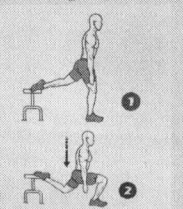

Perform split squat on one leg, elevated rear foot.

1. Stand a few feet in front of a bench or elevated surface.
2. Place your right foot behind you on the bench.
3. Lower your hips into a squat, keeping your left knee over your ankle.
4. Push through your left heel to return to the starting position.
5. Repeat on the other leg, alternating sides.

Single Leg Squat

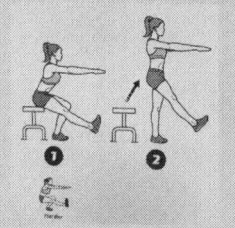

Stand on one leg, squat, maintain balance.

1. Stand on your right leg, extending your left leg in front.
2. Lower your hips into a squat, keeping your left leg elevated.
3. Maintain balance and keep your chest up.
4. Push through your right heel to return to the starting position.
5. Repeat on the other leg, alternating sides.

Skater Squat

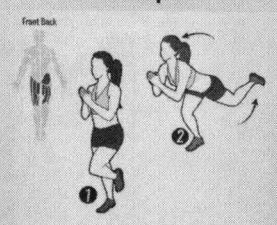

Balance on one leg, squat, touch opposite hand to foot.

1. Balance on your right leg, bending your left knee.
2. Lower into a squat while reaching your left hand towards your right foot.
3. Keep your back straight and chest up.
4. Push through your right heel to return to the starting position.
5. Repeat on the other leg, alternating sides.

Spiderman

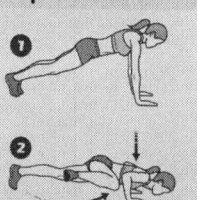

Bring knee to elbow during push-up, switch sides.

1. Start in a push-up position with hands under shoulders.
2. Lower your body towards the ground while bringing your right knee to your right elbow.
3. Push back up to the starting position.
4. Repeat with the left knee to the left elbow, alternating sides.
5. Continue for the desired number of repetitions.

Squat

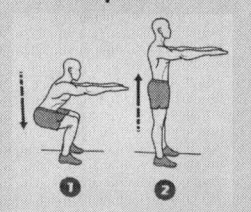

Stand, bend knees to lower body, keep back straight.

1. Stand with feet shoulder-width apart and arms extended in front.
2. Bend your knees and lower your hips into a squat.
3. Keep your back straight and chest up.
4. Push through your heels to return to the starting position.
5. Repeat for the desired number of repetitions.

Star Plank

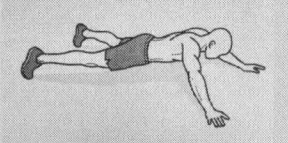

Extend arms and legs out from body in plank position.

1. Start in a plank position with hands under shoulders and feet together.
2. Extend your right arm and left leg out to the sides.
3. Hold for a moment, keeping your core engaged.
4. Return to the starting position and repeat with the left arm and right leg.
5. Alternate sides for the desired number of repetitions.

Step Up

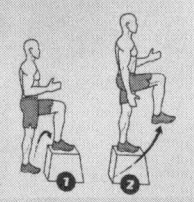

Step onto a raised platform, alternate legs.

1. Stand in front of a raised platform or bench.
2. Step up with your right foot, bringing your left knee towards your chest.
3. Step back down with your left foot, then your right foot.
4. Repeat with the left foot leading, alternating sides.
5. Continue for the desired number of repetitions.

Stretching

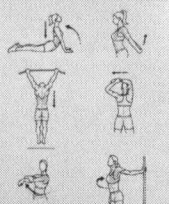

Perform various stretches to improve flexibility and cool down.

1. Perform a variety of stretches, targeting all major muscle groups.
2. Hold each stretch for 15-30 seconds.
3. Focus on slow, controlled movements to increase flexibility.
4. Include stretches for the hamstrings, quadriceps, calves, chest, back, and shoulders.
5. Ensure a thorough cool-down to aid in recovery.

Sumo Squat

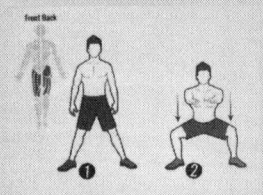

Wide stance squat, toes pointed out, lower body.

1. Stand with feet wider than shoulder-width apart and toes pointed out.
2. Lower your hips into a squat, keeping your back straight and chest up.
3. Ensure your knees track over your toes.
4. Push through your heels to return to the starting position.
5. Repeat for the desired number of repetitions.

Superman

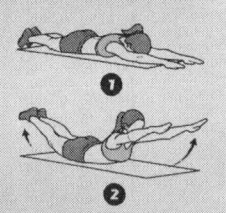

Extend arms and legs while face down, hold position.

1. Lie face down on the ground with arms extended forward and legs straight.
2. Lift your arms, chest, and legs off the ground simultaneously.
3. Hold the top position for a few seconds.
4. Lower back down to the starting position.
5. Repeat for the desired number of repetitions.

Swimmer

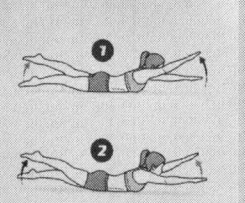

Lie face down, alternate lifting arms and legs.

1. Lie face down on the ground with arms extended forward and legs straight.
2. Lift your right arm and left leg off the ground simultaneously.
3. Lower them back down and lift your left arm and right leg.
4. Continue alternating sides in a swimming motion.
5. Repeat for the desired number of repetitions or time.

Tricep Dip

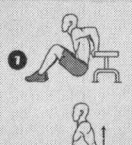

Dip body between bars, focus on triceps.

1. Sit on the edge of a bench or chair with hands gripping the edge.
2. Slide your hips off the edge, supporting your weight with your arms.
3. Lower your body by bending your elbows to a 90-degree angle.
4. Push through your palms to return to the starting position.
5. Repeat for the desired number of repetitions.

Tricep Push Up

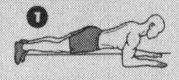

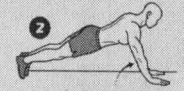

Push-up with hands under shoulders, elbows tight.

1. Start in a plank position with hands under shoulders and elbows close to your body.
2. Lower your body towards the ground, keeping elbows tight to your sides.
3. Push through your palms to return to the starting position.
4. Keep your body in a straight line throughout the movement.
5. Repeat for the desired number of repetitions.

Tuck Jumps

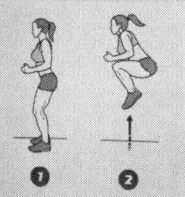

Jump high, tuck knees to chest mid-air.

1. Stand with feet hip-width apart and knees slightly bent.
2. Jump explosively, bringing your knees towards your chest.
3. Land softly on the balls of your feet with knees slightly bent.
4. Immediately jump again, maintaining quick, controlled movements.
5. Repeat for the desired number of repetitions or time.

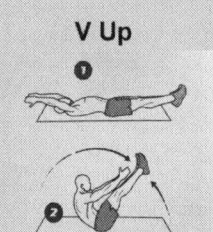

V Up

Lie back, lift legs and torso simultaneously, form 'V'.

1. Lie on your back with arms extended overhead and legs straight.
2. Simultaneously lift your legs and torso off the ground, reaching your hands towards your feet.
3. Form a "V" shape with your body at the top of the movement.
4. Lower back down to the starting position with control.
5. Repeat for the desired number of repetitions.

Walking Lunge

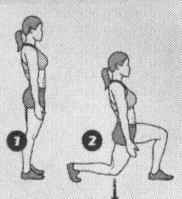

Step forward into a lunge, move forward alternating legs.

1. Stand with feet hip-width apart and hands on your hips.
2. Step forward with your right leg, lowering into a lunge.
3. Push through your right heel to stand and bring your left leg forward into the next lunge.
4. Continue alternating legs, moving forward with each step.
5. Repeat for the desired number of repetitions or distance.

Walking Toe Touches

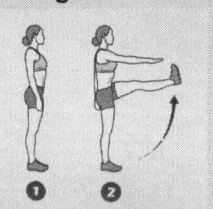

Walk, reach down to touch toes with opposite hand.

1. Stand with feet hip-width apart.
2. Step forward with your right leg, lifting it straight in front of you.
3. Reach your left hand to touch your right toes.
4. Lower your leg and step forward with your left leg, reaching your right hand to your left toes.
5. Continue alternating sides as you walk forward.

Wall Sit

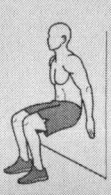

Sit against wall, legs at 90 degrees, hold position.

1. Stand with your back against a wall.
2. Slide down the wall until your thighs are parallel to the ground.
3. Keep your feet shoulder-width apart and knees at a 90-degree angle.
4. Hold this position for the desired amount of time.
5. Maintain tension in your thighs and keep your back flat against the wall.

Wall Squat

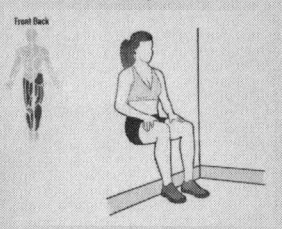

Lie face down, alternate lifting arms and legs.

1. Stand with your back against a wall, feet shoulder-width apart.
2. Slide down into a squat position, keeping your back against the wall.
3. Ensure your thighs are parallel to the ground and knees are above your ankles.
4. Hold this position for the desired time.
5. Maintain proper form by keeping your back straight and core engaged.

Wide/Narrow Push Up

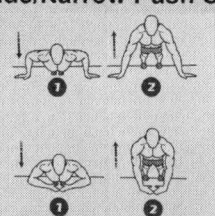

Perform push-ups with varying hand widths.

1. Start in a plank position with hands wider than shoulder-width apart.
2. Lower your body to the ground by bending your elbows.
3. Push through your palms to return to the starting position.
4. Move your hands closer together, directly under your shoulders.
5. Perform another push-up in this narrow position.
6. Alternate between wide and narrow push-ups for the desired repetitions.

Windshield Wiper

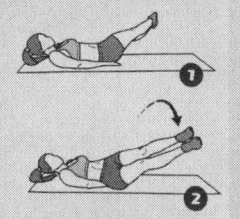

Swing legs side-to-side lying down, mimic wiper.

1. Lie on your back with arms extended out to the sides for support.
2. Lift your legs off the ground and bring them to a 90-degree angle.
3. Slowly lower your legs to the right side, keeping them together.
4. Bring your legs back to the center.
5. Lower your legs to the left side.
6. Continue alternating sides, mimicking a windshield wiper motion.

Dumbbell Exercises Guide

Dumbbell Exercises

ALTERNATING FRONT RAISE

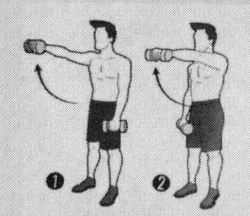

1. Stand with feet shoulder-width apart, holding a dumbbell in each hand, palms facing down.
2. Raise the right dumbbell to shoulder height, keeping the arm straight.
3. Lower the right dumbbell while simultaneously raising the left dumbbell to shoulder height.
4. Continue alternating arms for the desired number of repetitions.

Lift dumbbells alternately to shoulder height, palms down.

BENCH PRESS

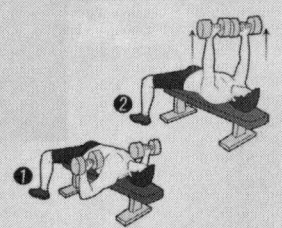

1. Lie on a flat bench with a dumbbell in each hand, feet flat on the floor.
2. Position the dumbbells near your chest, elbows bent at a 90-degree angle.
3. Press the dumbbells upward until your arms are fully extended above your chest.
4. Lower the dumbbells back to the starting position with control.
5. Repeat for the desired number of repetitions.

Push dumbbells up from chest while lying on a bench.

BOW EXTENSION

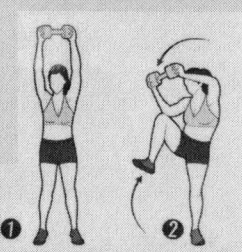

1. Stand with feet shoulder-width apart, holding a dumbbell in each hand.
2. Raise the dumbbells above your head, arms fully extended.
3. Pull the right dumbbell back as if drawing a bow, keeping the left arm extended.
4. Return the right dumbbell to the starting position and repeat with the left arm.
5. Alternate arms for the desired number of repetitions.

Pull dumbbell back like drawing a bow, alternating arms.

CALF RAISE

1. Stand with feet shoulder-width apart, holding a dumbbell in each hand.
2. Rise onto your toes as high as possible, keeping your core engaged.
3. Hold the top position briefly, then lower your heels back to the ground slowly.
4. Repeat for the desired number of repetitions.

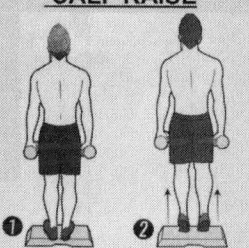

Rise onto toes holding dumbbells, lower slowly for calf work.

CHEST FLY

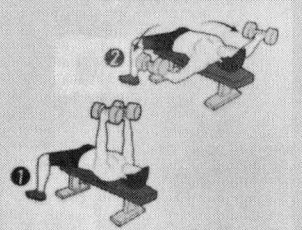

Extend arms wide on bench, bring dumbbells together above chest.

1. Lie on a flat bench with a dumbbell in each hand, arms extended above your chest, palms facing each other.
2. Slowly lower the dumbbells out to the sides, maintaining a slight bend in your elbows.
3. Lower until you feel a stretch in your chest.
4. Bring the dumbbells back together above your chest, squeezing your chest muscles.
5. Repeat for the desired number of repetitions.

CONCENTRATION CURL

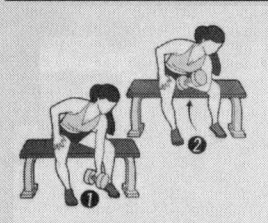

Curl dumbbell with elbow on thigh, focus on bicep.

1. Sit on a bench with feet flat on the floor, holding a dumbbell in your right hand.
2. Rest your right elbow on the inside of your right thigh, arm fully extended.
3. Curl the dumbbell toward your shoulder, keeping your upper arm stationary.
4. Squeeze your bicep at the top of the movement.
5. Lower the dumbbell back to the starting position with control.
6. Repeat for the desired number of repetitions, then switch arms.

DUMBBELL PULLOVER

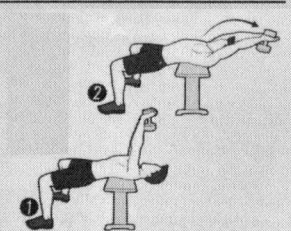

Lie on bench, swing dumbbell over head to chest level.

1. Lie on a flat bench, feet flat on the floor, holding a dumbbell with both hands above your chest.
2. Keeping your arms slightly bent, lower the dumbbell back over your head until you feel a stretch in your chest.
3. Pull the dumbbell back over your chest using your chest and back muscles.
4. Repeat for the desired number of repetitions.

FARMER'S WALK

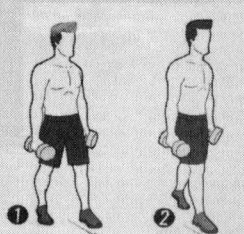

Walk holding heavy dumbbells at sides, maintain upright posture.

1. Stand with feet shoulder-width apart, holding a heavy dumbbell in each hand at your sides.
2. Maintain an upright posture with shoulders back and core engaged.
3. Walk forward for a specified distance or time, keeping your back straight and head up.
4. Turn around and walk back to the starting point if needed.
5. Repeat as necessary for the desired duration or distance.

FLOOR T RAISE

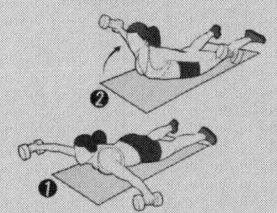

Lie face-down, lift dumbbells sideways forming a 'T'.

1. Lie face-down on the floor with arms extended to the sides, holding a dumbbell in each hand.
2. Lift the dumbbells up, forming a "T" shape with your body, squeezing your shoulder blades together.
3. Hold briefly at the top, then lower the dumbbells back to the floor.
4. Repeat for the desired number of repetitions.

GLUTE BRIDGE

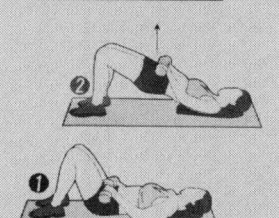

Press hips up while holding dumbbells, lying on floor.

1. Lie on your back with knees bent, feet flat on the floor, and a dumbbell held over your hips.
2. Press through your heels to lift your hips toward the ceiling, squeezing your glutes at the top.
3. Hold briefly, then lower your hips back to the floor.
4. Repeat for the desired number of repetitions.

GOBLET SQUAT

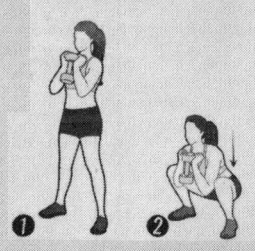

Squat holding dumbbell at chest with both hands.

1. Stand with feet shoulder-width apart, holding a dumbbell at chest level with both hands.
2. Squat down by bending your knees and hips, keeping your chest up and back straight.
3. Lower until your thighs are parallel to the floor, then push through your heels to return to standing.
4. Repeat for the desired number of repetitions.

GRIP CURL

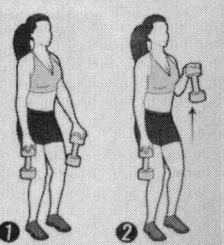

Curl dumbbells with palms facing each other, focus on forearms.

1. Stand with feet shoulder-width apart, holding a dumbbell in each hand, palms facing each other.
2. Curl the dumbbells toward your shoulders, focusing on using your forearms.
3. Squeeze your forearms at the top of the movement.
4. Lower the dumbbells back to the starting position with control.
5. Repeat for the desired number of repetitions.

HAMMER CURL

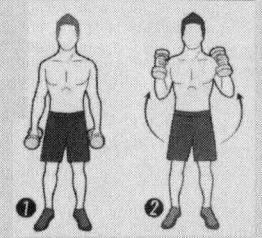

Curl dumbbells with thumbs up, emphasizing forearms.

1. Stand with feet shoulder-width apart, holding a dumbbell in each hand, palms facing your body.
2. Curl the dumbbells toward your shoulders, keeping your palms facing each other throughout the movement.
3. Squeeze your biceps at the top, then lower the dumbbells back to the starting position.
4. Repeat for the desired number of repetitions.

INCLINE BENCH PRESS

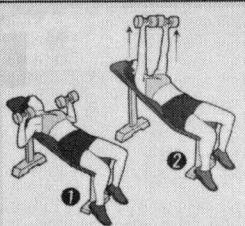

Press dumbbells from chest on inclined bench.

1. Lie on an incline bench with a dumbbell in each hand, feet flat on the floor.
2. Position the dumbbells near your chest, elbows bent at a 90-degree angle.
3. Press the dumbbells upward until your arms are fully extended above your chest.
4. Lower the dumbbells back to the starting position with control.
5. Repeat for the desired number of repetitions.

INCLINE ROW

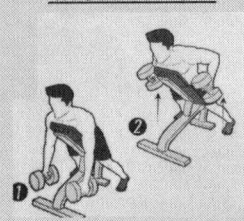

Pull dumbbells towards waist, bent over inclined bench.

1. Lie face-down on an incline bench with a dumbbell in each hand.
2. Pull the dumbbells toward your waist, squeezing your shoulder blades together.
3. Hold briefly at the top, then lower the dumbbells back to the starting position.
4. Repeat for the desired number of repetitions.

JUMP SQUAT

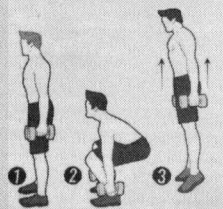

Perform explosive squats holding dumbbells for added resistance.

1. Stand with feet shoulder-width apart, holding a dumbbell in each hand.
2. Lower into a squat position by bending your knees and hips.
3. Explode upward into a jump, pushing through your heels.
4. Land softly and immediately lower back into a squat.
5. Repeat for the desired number of repetitions.

PLANK T

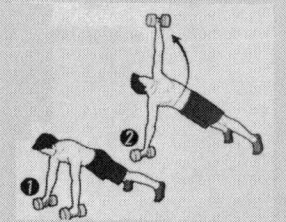

Hold plank and rotate lifting dumbbell in a 'T' pose.

1. Begin in a plank position, feet shoulder-width apart, holding a dumbbell in each hand.
2. Rotate your body to the right, lifting the right dumbbell towards the ceiling, forming a "T" shape with your body.
3. Return to the plank position and repeat on the left side.
4. Alternate sides for the desired number of repetitions.

RENEGADE ROW

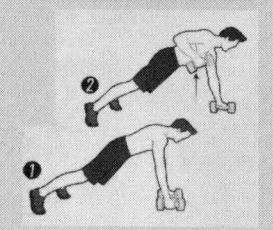

1. Start in a plank position with feet wide apart, holding a dumbbell in each hand.
2. Row the right dumbbell towards your hip, keeping your core stable and body straight.
3. Lower the right dumbbell and repeat with the left arm.
4. Alternate arms for the desired number of repetitions.

REVERSE FLY

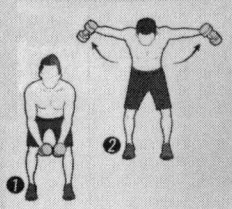

1. Stand with feet shoulder-width apart, knees slightly bent, holding a dumbbell in each hand.
2. Bend forward at the hips, keeping your back straight and arms hanging down.
3. Raise the dumbbells out to the sides, squeezing your shoulder blades together.
4. Lower the dumbbells back to the starting position.
5. Repeat for the desired number of repetitions.

REVERSE LUNGE

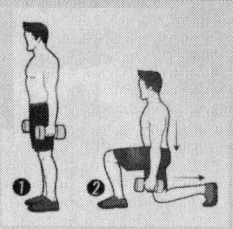

1. Stand with feet shoulder-width apart, holding a dumbbell in each hand.
2. Step back with your right foot, lowering your body until your left thigh is parallel to the floor.
3. Push through your left heel to return to the starting position.
4. Alternate legs for the desired number of repetitions.

ROMANIAN DEADLIFT

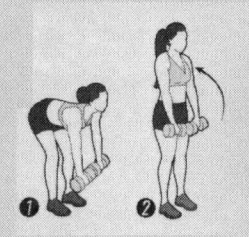

1. Stand with feet hip-width apart, holding a dumbbell in each hand.
2. Keep your knees slightly bent and back straight, hinge at the hips to lower the dumbbells down your legs.
3. Lower until you feel a stretch in your hamstrings, then return to the starting position by extending your hips.
4. Repeat for the desired number of repetitions.

RUSSIAN TWIST

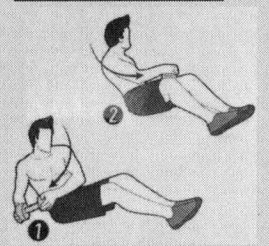

1. Sit on the floor with knees bent, holding a dumbbell with both hands.
2. Lean back slightly and lift your feet off the floor.
3. Twist your torso to the right, touching the dumbbell to the floor beside you.
4. Twist to the left, repeating the movement on the opposite side.
5. Alternate sides for the desired number of repetitions.

Sit and twist holding dumbbell, touch alternating sides.

SEESAW ROW

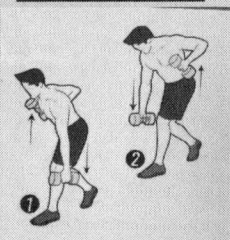

1. Stand with feet shoulder-width apart, holding a dumbbell in each hand.
2. Bend forward at the hips, keeping your back straight and arms hanging down.
3. Row the right dumbbell towards your waist while lowering the left dumbbell.
4. Alternate arms, mimicking a seesaw motion.
5. Repeat for the desired number of repetitions.

Alternate rowing dumbbells while bent over, mimicking a seesaw.

SHOULDER PRESS

1. Stand with feet shoulder-width apart, holding a dumbbell in each hand at shoulder height, palms facing forward.
2. Press the dumbbells overhead until your arms are fully extended.
3. Lower the dumbbells back to shoulder height with control.
4. Repeat for the desired number of repetitions.

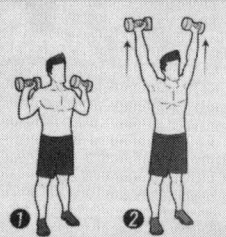

Press dumbbells overhead from shoulders, palms facing forward.

SHOULDER SHRUG

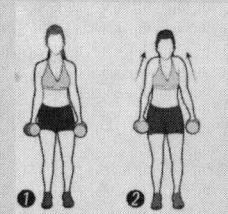

Lift shoulders to ears holding dumbbells, lower slowly.

1. Stand with feet shoulder-width apart, holding a dumbbell in each hand at your sides.
2. Lift your shoulders towards your ears, keeping your arms straight.
3. Hold for a brief moment at the top.
4. Slowly lower your shoulders back to the starting position.
5. Repeat for the desired number of repetitions.

SIDE BEND

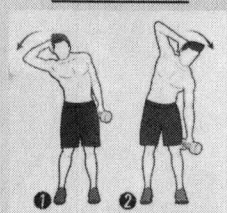

Bend sideways holding dumbbell, return to upright position.

1. Stand with feet shoulder-width apart, holding a dumbbell in your right hand.
2. Place your left hand on your hip and bend to the right, lowering the dumbbell toward your knee.
3. Return to the upright position.
4. Perform the desired number of repetitions, then switch sides and repeat.

SIDE LUNGE

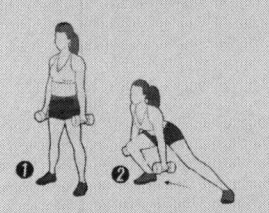

Step to the side into a lunge, holding dumbbells.

1. Stand with feet together, holding a dumbbell in each hand.
2. Step your right foot out to the side, bending your right knee and keeping your left leg straight.
3. Lower your body into a lunge position, keeping your chest up.
4. Push through your right foot to return to the starting position.
5. Alternate sides for the desired number of repetitions.

SIDE RAISE

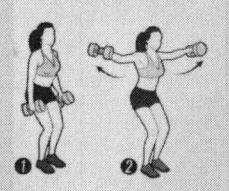

Lift dumbbells sideways to shoulder level, palms down.

1. Stand with feet shoulder-width apart, holding a dumbbell in each hand at your sides, palms facing your body.
2. Raise the dumbbells out to the sides until they reach shoulder height, keeping a slight bend in your elbows.
3. Lower the dumbbells back to the starting position with control.
4. Repeat for the desired number of repetitions.

SINGLE ARM ROW

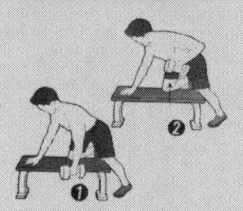

Pull dumbbell back while bent over, switch arms.

1. Place your left knee and hand on a bench, holding a dumbbell in your right hand.
2. Keep your back straight and pull the dumbbell towards your waist, squeezing your shoulder blade.
3. Lower the dumbbell back to the starting position with control.
4. Perform the desired number of repetitions, then switch sides and repeat.

STEP-UP

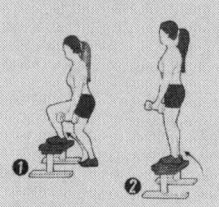

Step onto a bench holding dumbbells, alternate legs.

1. Stand facing a bench, holding a dumbbell in each hand.
2. Step onto the bench with your right foot, pressing through your heel to lift your body up.
3. Step down with your left foot, then your right.
4. Alternate legs for the desired number of repetitions.

SUMO SQUAT

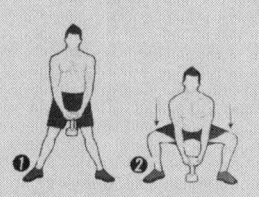

Wide stance squat holding a dumbbell with both hands.

1. Stand with feet wider than shoulder-width apart, toes pointing outward, holding a dumbbell with both hands in front of you.
2. Squat down by bending your knees and hips, keeping your chest up and back straight.
3. Lower until your thighs are parallel to the floor, then push through your heels to return to standing.
4. Repeat for the desired number of repetitions.

SWING

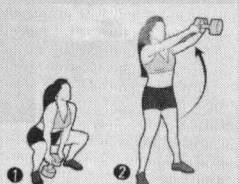

Swing dumbbell between legs to chest level, hinge at hips.

1. Stand with feet shoulder-width apart, holding a dumbbell with both hands.
2. Hinge at your hips, swinging the dumbbell between your legs.
3. Thrust your hips forward to swing the dumbbell up to chest level.
4. Let the dumbbell swing back down between your legs and repeat.
5. Perform for the desired number of repetitions.

THRUSTER

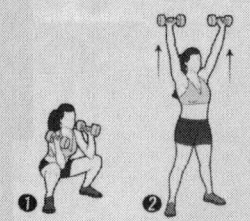

Squat with dumbbells at shoulders, press up while standing.

1. Stand with feet shoulder-width apart, holding dumbbells at your shoulders.
2. Lower into a squat by bending your knees and hips.
3. Push through your heels to stand up while pressing the dumbbells overhead.
4. Lower the dumbbells back to your shoulders and repeat.
5. Perform for the desired number of repetitions.

TRICEP EXTENSION

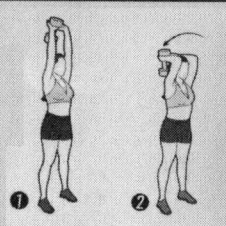

Extend dumbbells overhead, focus on tricep contraction.

1. Stand with feet shoulder-width apart, holding a dumbbell with both hands overhead.
2. Keep your elbows close to your head and lower the dumbbell behind your neck.
3. Extend your arms to lift the dumbbell back overhead, focusing on tricep contraction.
4. Repeat for the desired number of repetitions.

TRICEP KICKBACK

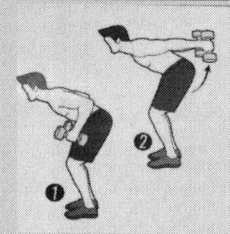

Lean over, extend dumbbell back from bent elbow.

1. Stand with feet hip-width apart, holding a dumbbell in each hand.
2. Bend forward at the hips, keeping your back straight and elbows bent at 90 degrees.
3. Extend your arms backward, straightening your elbows and squeezing your triceps.
4. Return to the starting position with control.
5. Repeat for the desired number of repetitions.

V-SIT CROSS JAB

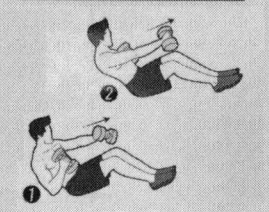

Sit, twist and jab with dumbbells across the body.

1. Sit on the floor with knees bent, holding a dumbbell in each hand.
2. Lean back slightly and lift your feet off the ground.
3. Twist your torso to the right, jabbing the left dumbbell across your body.
4. Repeat on the left side, jabbing with the right dumbbell.
5. Alternate sides for the desired number of repetitions.

V-UP

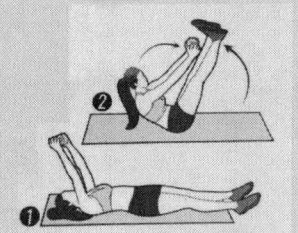

Lie back, lift legs and torso simultaneously holding dumbbell.

1. Lie on your back with arms extended overhead, holding a dumbbell.
2. Simultaneously lift your legs and torso, bringing the dumbbell towards your feet.
3. Keep your arms and legs straight throughout the movement.
4. Lower your body back to the starting position with control.
5. Repeat for the desired number of repetitions.

WOODCHOP

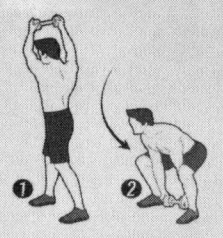

Swing dumbbell diagonally across body, squat to lift and lower.

1. Stand with feet shoulder-width apart, holding a dumbbell with both hands.
2. Squat down, bringing the dumbbell diagonally across your body to the outside of one knee.
3. Stand up, swinging the dumbbell diagonally across your body to above your opposite shoulder.
4. Return to the squat position and repeat.
5. Alternate sides for the desired number of repetitions.

WRIST CURL

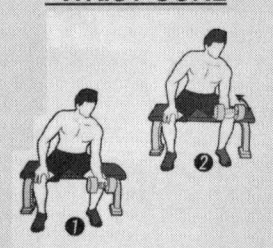

Curl wrist upward holding dumbbells, focus on forearm muscles.

1. Sit on a bench, holding a dumbbell in each hand with palms facing up.
2. Rest your forearms on your thighs, letting your wrists hang over the edge.
3. Curl your wrists upward, lifting the dumbbells.
4. Lower the dumbbells back to the starting position with control.
5. Repeat for the desired number of repetitions.

Kettlebell Exercises Guide

Kettlebell Exercises

ALTERNATING CURL

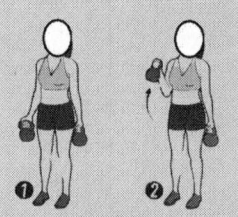

Curl kettlebells alternately, focus on bicep isolation.

1. Stand with feet shoulder-width apart, holding a kettlebell in each hand.
2. Keep your elbows close to your torso and your palms facing forward.
3. Curl the right kettlebell while keeping the left arm stationary.
4. Lower the right kettlebell back to the starting position.
5. Repeat the movement with the left kettlebell.
6. Continue alternating curls, focusing on bicep isolation.

AROUND THE BODY

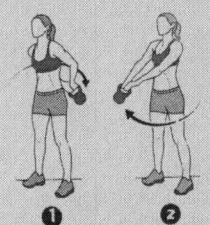

Pass kettlebell around body, maintain core control.

1. Stand with feet hip-width apart, holding a kettlebell in front of you.
2. Pass the kettlebell around your body, starting from the front.
3. Keep your core engaged to maintain balance.
4. Transfer the kettlebell from one hand to the other behind your back.
5. Continue the motion, passing the kettlebell around your body in a circular motion.
6. Reverse the direction halfway through the set.

ATLAS SWING

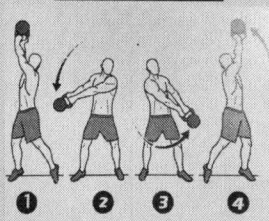

Swing kettlebell up, catch at chest level.

1. Stand with feet shoulder-width apart, holding a kettlebell in one hand.
2. Swing the kettlebell between your legs.
3. Drive your hips forward to swing the kettlebell up to chest level.
4. Catch the kettlebell with your other hand at chest height.
5. Swing the kettlebell back down and repeat the motion.
6. Switch hands after completing the set.

BENT OVER ROW

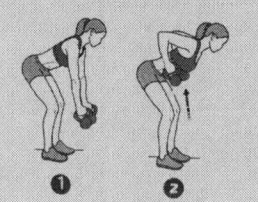

Hinge forward, row kettlebell to hip, switch sides.

1. Stand with feet hip-width apart, holding a kettlebell in each hand.
2. Hinge forward at the hips, keeping your back straight.
3. Let the kettlebells hang directly under your shoulders.
4. Row the right kettlebell to your hip, squeezing your shoulder blade.
5. Lower the right kettlebell and repeat with the left kettlebell.
6. Alternate sides, maintaining a controlled movement.

BOB AND WEAVE

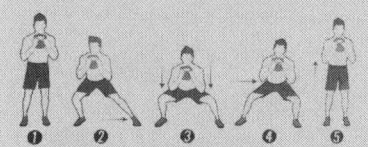

Duck and weave sideways holding kettlebell.

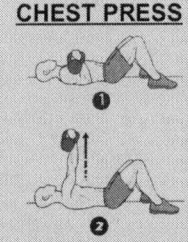

1. Stand with feet shoulder-width apart, holding a kettlebell with both hands.
2. Bend your knees slightly and engage your core.
3. Duck down to the right, keeping the kettlebell close to your chest.
4. Weave under an imaginary obstacle, moving to the left.
5. Stand up on the left side and repeat the movement to the right.
6. Continue ducking and weaving, maintaining a smooth rhythm.

CHEST PRESS

Press kettlebell from chest while lying down.

1. Lie on your back with your knees bent and feet flat on the floor.
2. Hold a kettlebell in each hand, with your elbows bent and close to your body.
3. Press the kettlebells straight up, extending your arms fully.
4. Lower the kettlebells back down to your chest.
5. Keep your movements controlled and your core engaged.
6. Repeat the press, focusing on chest muscle engagement.

CLEAN

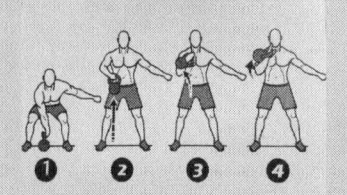

Lift kettlebell to shoulder, flip grip at top.

1. Stand with feet shoulder-width apart, holding a kettlebell in one hand.
2. Bend your knees and lower the kettlebell between your legs.
3. Drive through your heels and extend your hips to pull the kettlebell up.
4. Flip your grip at the top, catching the kettlebell on the back of your wrist.
5. Lower the kettlebell back down to the starting position.
6. Repeat the movement, focusing on a smooth, controlled lift.

CURL

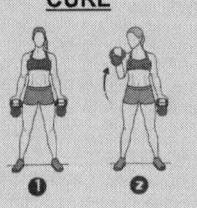

Curl kettlebell using standard grip, focus on biceps.

1. Stand with feet shoulder-width apart, holding a kettlebell in each hand.
2. Keep your elbows close to your torso and your palms facing inward.
3. Curl both kettlebells simultaneously, focusing on your biceps.
4. Lower the kettlebells back to the starting position.
5. Maintain a controlled movement throughout the exercise.
6. Repeat the curls, ensuring full range of motion.

DEADLIFT

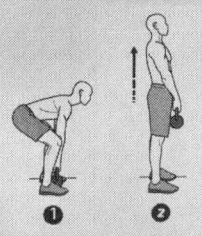

Lift kettlebell from ground, keep back straight.

1. Stand with feet hip-width apart, kettlebell on the floor between your feet.
2. Hinge at your hips and bend your knees to grasp the kettlebell handle.
3. Keep your back straight, engage your core, and drive through your heels to lift the kettlebell.
4. Stand up fully, keeping the kettlebell close to your body.
5. Reverse the movement to lower the kettlebell back to the ground.
6. Repeat, ensuring proper form throughout.

DECK SQUAT

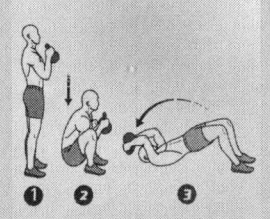

Squat, roll back, stand up while holding kettlebell.

1. Stand with feet shoulder-width apart, holding a kettlebell close to your chest.
2. Squat down and roll back onto your back, tucking your knees towards your chest.
3. Use momentum to roll forward and stand back up, maintaining the kettlebell at your chest.
4. Keep your core engaged to assist with the movement.
5. Repeat the squat and roll sequence.
6. Focus on smooth transitions between the rolling and standing phases.

DEFICIT PUSH UP

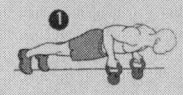

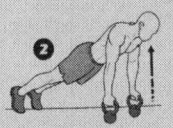

Push-up holding kettlebell to increase depth.

1. Place two kettlebells on the floor shoulder-width apart.
2. Assume a push-up position with hands gripping the kettlebell handles.
3. Lower your body until your chest is in line with the kettlebells.
4. Push through your palms to return to the starting position.
5. Keep your body in a straight line from head to heels.
6. Repeat, maintaining a controlled pace and proper form.

DOUBLE ARM SWING

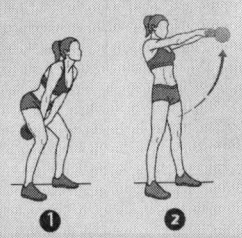

Swing kettlebell with both hands, hinge at hips.

1. Stand with feet shoulder-width apart, holding a kettlebell with both hands.
2. Hinge at your hips, letting the kettlebell swing back between your legs.
3. Drive your hips forward to swing the kettlebell up to shoulder height.
4. Keep your arms straight but relaxed throughout the movement.
5. Allow the kettlebell to swing back down between your legs.
6. Repeat, maintaining a fluid motion.

FARMER'S WALK

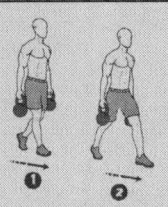

Walk holding kettlebell in each hand, keep back straight.

1. Stand with feet shoulder-width apart, holding a kettlebell in each hand.
2. Engage your core and keep your back straight.
3. Walk forward, maintaining an upright posture.
4. Keep the kettlebells at your sides with your arms straight.
5. Walk for the desired distance or time.
6. Focus on steady, controlled steps.

FIGURE EIGHT

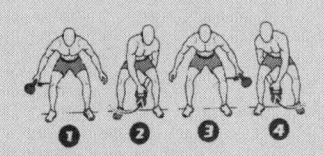

Pass kettlebell through legs in figure-eight motion.

1. Stand with feet wider than shoulder-width apart, holding a kettlebell in one hand.
2. Bend your knees and hinge at your hips to pass the kettlebell between your legs.
3. Grab the kettlebell with the opposite hand behind your leg.
4. Swing the kettlebell around the outside of your leg and pass it through your legs again.
5. Continue the figure-eight motion, alternating hands.
6. Keep your core engaged and maintain a stable stance.

FRONT RAISE

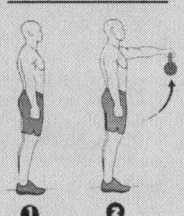

Lift kettlebell to shoulder, flip grip at top.

1. Stand with feet shoulder-width apart, holding a kettlebell in one hand.
2. Keep your arm straight and lift the kettlebell to shoulder height.
3. Flip your grip at the top, rotating the kettlebell.
4. Lower the kettlebell back to the starting position.
5. Repeat the movement, maintaining a controlled pace.
6. Switch hands and repeat for the other side.

GOBLET SQUAT

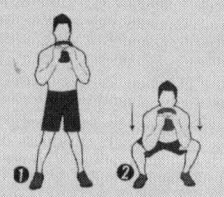

Squat holding kettlebell close to chest.

1. Stand with feet shoulder-width apart, holding a kettlebell close to your chest with both hands.
2. Engage your core and squat down, keeping your chest up and back straight.
3. Lower your hips until your thighs are parallel to the ground.
4. Drive through your heels to return to the standing position.
5. Keep the kettlebell close to your chest throughout the movement.
6. Repeat, maintaining proper squat form.

GOOD MORNING

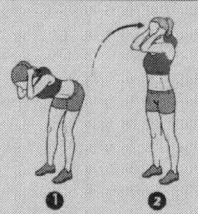

Hinge at hips holding kettlebell, focus on hamstrings.

1. Stand with feet shoulder-width apart, holding a kettlebell close to your chest.
2. Hinge at your hips, keeping your back straight and knees slightly bent.
3. Lower your torso until it is parallel to the ground.
4. Engage your hamstrings and glutes to return to the standing position.
5. Keep the kettlebell stable and your core engaged throughout the movement.
6. Repeat, maintaining proper form to avoid strain on your lower back.

HALF TURKISH GET UP

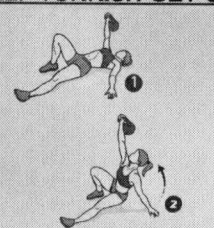

Rise from floor to seated, kettlebell overhead.

1. Lie on your back with your right leg bent and right foot flat on the floor, holding a kettlebell in your right hand.
2. Extend your left arm and leg on the floor.
3. Press the kettlebell straight up, keeping your eyes on it.
4. Roll onto your left forearm, then onto your left hand.
5. Push through your right foot to lift your hips off the ground.
6. Come up to a seated position, maintaining the kettlebell overhead.
7. Reverse the steps to return to the starting position.
8. Repeat on the other side.

HALO

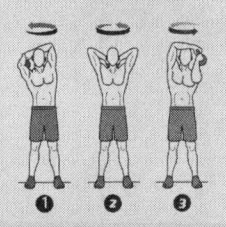

Circle kettlebell around head, maintain posture.

1. Stand with feet shoulder-width apart, holding a kettlebell by the horns at chest level.
2. Circle the kettlebell around your head, starting from the front.
3. Keep your core engaged and your head steady.
4. Complete the circle by bringing the kettlebell back to the starting position.
5. Perform the movement slowly and smoothly to avoid straining your neck.
6. Reverse the direction halfway through the set.

HIP BRIDGE PULLOVER

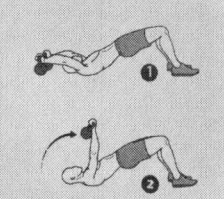

Hip thrust while pulling kettlebell over chest.

1. Lie on your back with your knees bent and feet flat on the floor, holding a kettlebell with both hands above your chest.
2. Lift your hips into a bridge position, engaging your glutes and core.
3. Slowly lower the kettlebell over your head until your arms are fully extended.
4. Pull the kettlebell back to the starting position above your chest.
5. Lower your hips back to the ground.
6. Repeat, maintaining a controlled movement throughout.

I LEG REV. PLANK

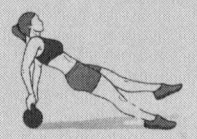

One-leg reverse plank, hold kettlebell above chest.

1. Sit on the floor with your legs extended and a kettlebell next to you.
2. Place your hands on the ground behind you and lift your hips into a reverse plank position.
3. Raise your right leg off the ground and hold the kettlebell above your chest with both hands.
4. Keep your body in a straight line from head to the left heel.
5. Hold the position for the desired amount of time.
6. Lower your leg and hips, then switch sides.

JUMP SWING

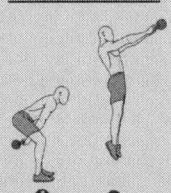

❶ ❷
Explosive swing with a jump at top of motion.

1. Stand with feet shoulder-width apart, holding a kettlebell with both hands.
2. Hinge at your hips, letting the kettlebell swing back between your legs.
3. Drive your hips forward and swing the kettlebell up to shoulder height.
4. At the top of the swing, explosively jump off the ground.
5. Land softly and allow the kettlebell to swing back down between your legs.
6. Repeat the movement, focusing on a smooth transition between the swing and jump.

L SIT & HOLD

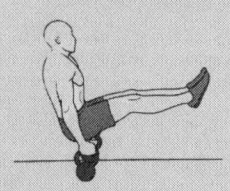

Sit, legs straight, hold kettlebell, maintain L-shape.

1. Sit on the ground with your legs extended straight in front of you.
2. Place a kettlebell on the ground between your legs.
3. Lift your legs and torso off the ground, forming an L shape with your body.
4. Hold the kettlebell with both hands above your chest.
5. Keep your core engaged and maintain the L shape.
6. Hold the position for the desired amount of time.

LEG RAISE

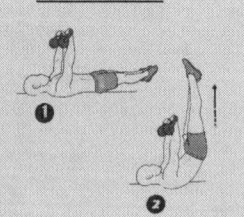

❶ ❷
Raise legs while lying down, hold kettlebell for weight.

1. Lie on your back with your legs extended and a kettlebell held in both hands above your chest.
2. Engage your core and lift your legs off the ground.
3. Raise your legs until they are perpendicular to the floor.
4. Slowly lower your legs back to the starting position without letting them touch the ground.
5. Keep the kettlebell stable and your lower back pressed into the floor.
6. Repeat, maintaining a controlled movement throughout.

LUNGE

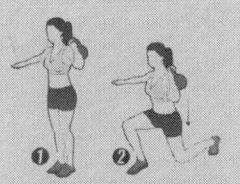

Hinge at hips holding kettlebell, focus on hamstrings.

1. Stand with feet shoulder-width apart, holding a kettlebell with both hands.
2. Step forward with your right foot and lower your hips, bending both knees to 90 degrees.
3. Keep your back straight and core engaged.
4. Push through your right heel to return to the starting position.
5. Repeat on the left leg.
6. Focus on keeping your weight evenly distributed and maintaining balance.

LUNGE PASS

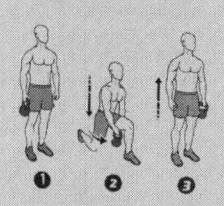

Pass kettlebell under leg during lunge.

1. Stand with feet hip-width apart, holding a kettlebell in your right hand.
2. Step forward with your left foot into a lunge position.
3. Pass the kettlebell under your left thigh to your left hand.
4. Push through your left heel to return to the starting position.
5. Repeat on the other side, passing the kettlebell under your right thigh.
6. Maintain a controlled motion, ensuring a stable core.

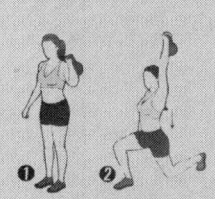

LUNGE PRESS

Lunge, press kettlebell overhead simultaneously.

1. Stand with feet shoulder-width apart, holding a kettlebell in your right hand.
2. Step forward with your left foot into a lunge position.
3. As you lower into the lunge, press the kettlebell overhead.
4. Keep your core engaged and back straight.
5. Push through your left heel to return to the starting position, lowering the kettlebell.
6. Repeat on the other side, ensuring synchronized movements.

OVERHEAD SIT UP

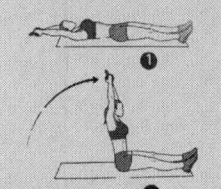

Sit-up with kettlebell held overhead.

1. Lie on your back with legs extended and a kettlebell held overhead with both hands.
2. Engage your core and sit up, keeping the kettlebell overhead.
3. Reach a seated position with your torso upright.
4. Slowly lower back down to the starting position.
5. Keep your arms extended and the kettlebell stable throughout the movement.
6. Repeat, focusing on a controlled ascent and descent.

OVERHEAD SQUAT

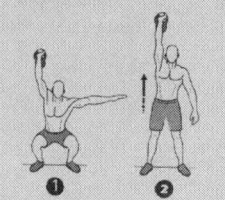

Squat with kettlebell held above head.

1. Stand with feet shoulder-width apart, holding a kettlebell overhead with both hands.
2. Engage your core and squat down, keeping the kettlebell stable.
3. Lower your hips until your thighs are parallel to the ground.
4. Push through your heels to return to the standing position.
5. Keep your back straight and chest up throughout the movement.
6. Repeat, ensuring the kettlebell remains overhead.

PISTOL SQUAT

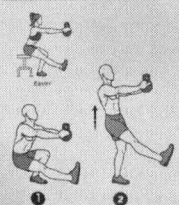

One-legged squat holding kettlebell for balance.

1. Stand on your right leg, holding a kettlebell in front of your chest with both hands.
2. Extend your left leg forward and lower into a one-legged squat.
3. Keep your chest up and core engaged.
4. Push through your right heel to return to the starting position.
5. Repeat on the left leg.
6. Focus on balance and control throughout the movement.

PLANK PULL THROUGH

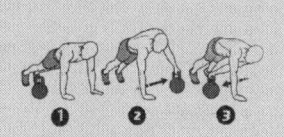

Plank, pull kettlebell across floor under chest.

1. Start in a plank position with a kettlebell to the right side of your body.
2. Reach your left hand under your body to pull the kettlebell across to the left side.
3. Return your left hand to the plank position.
4. Repeat with your right hand, pulling the kettlebell back to the right side.
5. Keep your core engaged and hips stable throughout the movement.
6. Continue alternating sides, maintaining a strong plank position.

PULLOVER

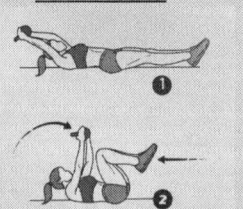

Lie back, pull kettlebell from overhead to chest.

1. Lie on your back with knees bent and feet flat on the floor, holding a kettlebell with both hands.
2. Extend your arms overhead, lowering the kettlebell towards the floor.
3. Engage your core and pull the kettlebell back over your chest.
4. Keep your arms slightly bent and the movement controlled.
5. Lower the kettlebell back to the starting position.
6. Repeat, focusing on a smooth, controlled motion.

PUSH-UP

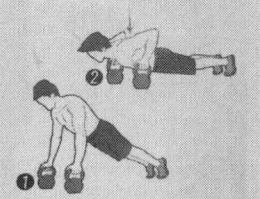

Standard push-up holding kettlebell handles.

1. Start in a plank position with hands gripping kettlebell handles.
2. Lower your body until your chest touches the ground, keeping elbows close to your body.
3. Engage your core and maintain a straight line from head to heels.
4. Push through your palms to return to the starting position.
5. Repeat, focusing on controlled movements and maintaining proper form.
6. Ensure your shoulders, hips, and feet stay aligned throughout.

RENEGADE

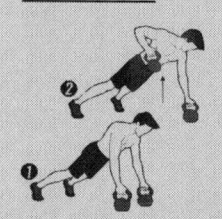

Plank and row kettlebells, alternating sides.

1. Start in a plank position with a kettlebell in each hand.
2. Row the right kettlebell to your hip while stabilizing your body with your left hand.
3. Lower the right kettlebell back to the ground.
4. Repeat the row with the left kettlebell.
5. Alternate sides, maintaining a strong plank position.
6. Keep your core engaged to prevent hip rotation.

RENEGADE ROW

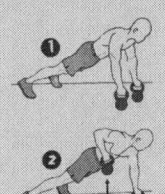

Row kettlebells alternately in plank position.

1. Assume a plank position with hands gripping kettlebell handles.
2. Row the right kettlebell to your hip, keeping your body stable.
3. Lower the right kettlebell back to the ground.
4. Repeat the row with the left kettlebell.
5. Alternate sides, maintaining a strong core.
6. Focus on controlled movements and avoid twisting your hips.

RUSSIAN TWIST

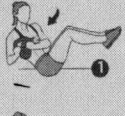

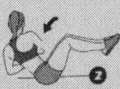

Twist torso holding kettlebell, seated on ground.

1. Sit on the ground with knees bent and feet flat, holding a kettlebell with both hands.
2. Lean back slightly to engage your core and lift your feet off the ground.
3. Twist your torso to the right, bringing the kettlebell beside your hip.
4. Twist to the left, bringing the kettlebell beside your left hip.
5. Continue alternating sides in a controlled motion.
6. Keep your back straight and core engaged throughout.

SHOULDER PRESS

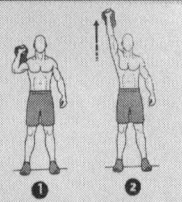

Press kettlebell overhead from shoulder level.

1. Stand with feet shoulder-width apart, holding a kettlebell in one hand at shoulder level.
2. Engage your core and press the kettlebell overhead until your arm is fully extended.
3. Lower the kettlebell back to shoulder level.
4. Repeat the press, maintaining a controlled movement.
5. Switch hands and repeat on the other side.
6. Focus on keeping your body stable and avoiding leaning.

SIDE BEND

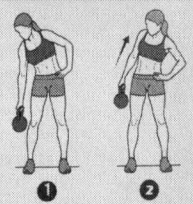

Bend sideways holding kettlebell, return upright.

1. Stand with feet shoulder-width apart, holding a kettlebell in your right hand.
2. Place your left hand on your hip and engage your core.
3. Bend sideways to the right, lowering the kettlebell towards your knee.
4. Return to the starting position by engaging your left obliques.
5. Repeat for the desired number of repetitions.
6. Switch sides and repeat the movement.

SIDE LUNGE

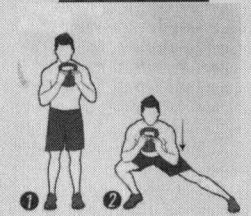

Step to side into lunge, kettlebell in hand for weight.

1. Stand with feet together, holding a kettlebell close to your chest.
2. Step to the right into a lunge, bending your right knee and keeping your left leg straight.
3. Push through your right heel to return to the starting position.
4. Repeat on the left side, stepping into a left lunge.
5. Alternate sides, maintaining a strong core and upright posture.
6. Focus on controlled movements and balance.

SIDE PLANK

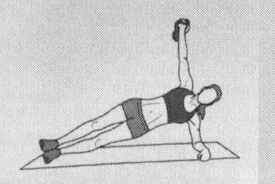

Hold side plank, lift kettlebell with free hand.

1. Start in a side plank position on your right elbow, with your body forming a straight line.
2. Hold a kettlebell in your left hand, resting it on your hip.
3. Lift the kettlebell towards the ceiling, keeping your arm straight.
4. Lower the kettlebell back to your hip.
5. Maintain the side plank position throughout the movement.
6. Switch sides and repeat the movement on the other side.

SIDE PLANK ROW

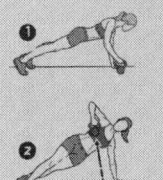

Row kettlebell in side plank position, stabilize core.

1. Start in a side plank position on your right elbow, body in a straight line.
2. Hold a kettlebell in your left hand, extended in front of you.
3. Engage your core and row the kettlebell towards your left hip.
4. Keep your body stable, avoiding any hip rotation.
5. Lower the kettlebell back to the starting position.
6. Repeat, then switch sides.

SIDE RAISE

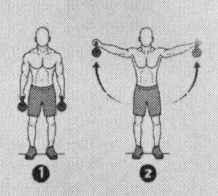

Lift kettlebell laterally to shoulder height.

1. Stand with feet shoulder-width apart, holding a kettlebell in each hand at your sides.
2. Engage your core and raise both kettlebells laterally to shoulder height.
3. Keep a slight bend in your elbows.
4. Lower the kettlebells back to the starting position.
5. Repeat, maintaining a controlled movement.
6. Avoid shrugging your shoulders during the raise.

SIDE SWING

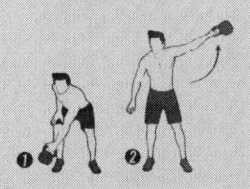

Swing kettlebell side to side, maintain grip.

1. Stand with feet shoulder-width apart, holding a kettlebell in your right hand.
2. Swing the kettlebell to your left side, pivoting on your feet.
3. Allow the kettlebell to swing back to the right side, pivoting your feet in the opposite direction.
4. Keep your core engaged and your movements controlled.
5. Repeat for the desired number of repetitions.
6. Switch hands and repeat the movement.

SIDEWINDER

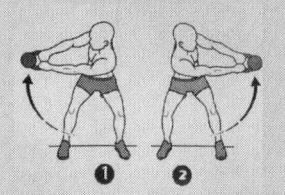

Move kettlebell in zigzag motion while holding squat.

1. Stand with feet wider than shoulder-width apart, holding a kettlebell with both hands.
2. Lower into a squat position, keeping your back straight.
3. Swing the kettlebell from side to side in a zigzag motion.
4. Maintain the squat position throughout the movement.
5. Keep your core engaged and movements smooth.
6. Repeat for the desired number of repetitions.

SINGLE ARM ROW

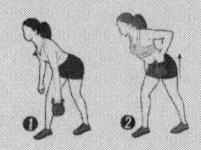

Row kettlebell with one arm, keep other hand free.

1. Stand with feet shoulder-width apart, holding a kettlebell in your right hand.
2. Hinge at your hips, keeping your back straight and knees slightly bent.
3. Row the kettlebell to your right hip, keeping your elbow close to your body.
4. Lower the kettlebell back to the starting position.
5. Repeat for the desired number of repetitions.
6. Switch hands and repeat the movement.

SINGLE ARM SWING

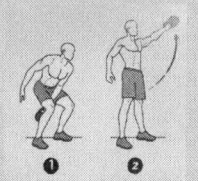

Swing kettlebell with one hand, switch hands mid-air.

1. Stand with feet shoulder-width apart, holding a kettlebell in your right hand.
2. Hinge at your hips, swinging the kettlebell back between your legs.
3. Drive your hips forward to swing the kettlebell up to shoulder height.
4. At the top of the swing, switch the kettlebell to your left hand.
5. Allow the kettlebell to swing back down between your legs.
6. Repeat, alternating hands at the top of each swing.

SINGLE LEG DEADLIFT

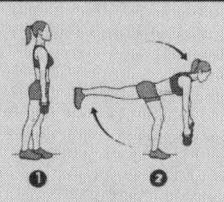

Deadlift on one leg holding kettlebell for balance.

1. Stand on your right leg, holding a kettlebell in your left hand.
2. Hinge at your hips, extending your left leg back and lowering the kettlebell towards the ground.
3. Keep your back straight and core engaged.
4. Return to the starting position by driving through your right heel.
5. Repeat for the desired number of repetitions.
6. Switch legs and repeat the movement.

SINGLE LEG ROW

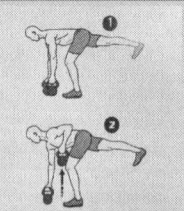

Row kettlebell while standing on one leg.

1. Stand on your right leg, holding a kettlebell in your left hand.
2. Hinge at your hips, extending your left leg back and lowering the kettlebell towards the ground.
3. Row the kettlebell to your left hip, keeping your back straight.
4. Lower the kettlebell back to the starting position.
5. Repeat for the desired number of repetitions.
6. Switch legs and repeat the movement.

SNATCH

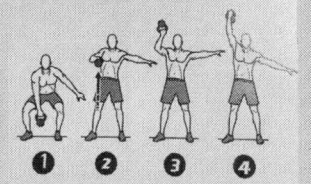

Lift kettlebell overhead in one motion, lock arm.

1. Stand with feet shoulder-width apart, a kettlebell between your feet.
2. Bend at the hips and knees to grab the kettlebell with one hand.
3. Explosively drive through your heels, pulling the kettlebell upwards.
4. As the kettlebell reaches chest height, flip your wrist and punch upward.
5. Lock your arm overhead, ensuring the kettlebell is stable.
6. Lower the kettlebell back to the starting position and repeat.

SQUAT

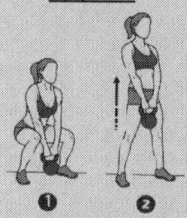

Squat holding kettlebell at chest or between legs.

1. Stand with feet shoulder-width apart, holding a kettlebell at chest level or between your legs.
2. Engage your core and squat down, pushing your hips back.
3. Lower your body until your thighs are parallel to the ground.
4. Keep your chest up and back straight throughout the movement.
5. Push through your heels to return to the starting position.
6. Repeat, maintaining proper form.

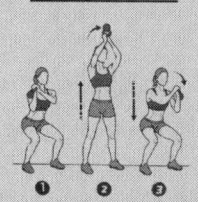

SQUAT FLIP

Squat, flip kettlebell at chest level during stand.

1. Stand with feet shoulder-width apart, holding a kettlebell at chest level.
2. Squat down, keeping the kettlebell stable.
3. As you stand up, flip the kettlebell at chest level, catching it with both hands.
4. Return to the starting position and repeat the movement.
5. Ensure the flip is controlled and smooth.
6. Focus on keeping your core engaged and back straight.

STRAIGHT ARM SIT

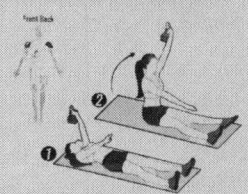

Sit-up with arms straight holding kettlebell.

1. Lie on your back with legs extended, holding a kettlebell with both hands above your chest.
2. Engage your core and sit up, keeping your arms extended straight.
3. Reach a seated position with the kettlebell above your head.
4. Slowly lower back down to the starting position.
5. Maintain straight arms and a stable kettlebell throughout the movement.
6. Repeat, focusing on controlled movements.

STRETCHING

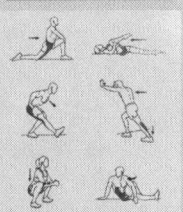

Use kettlebell for support or resistance during stretches.

1. Use a kettlebell for support or resistance during various stretches.
2. Perform seated stretches with the kettlebell for added resistance.
3. Use the kettlebell to assist in deepening your stretches.
4. Incorporate the kettlebell into dynamic stretches for improved flexibility.
5. Ensure each stretch is held for 20-30 seconds.
6. Repeat each stretch, focusing on maintaining proper form.

SUMO HIGH PULL

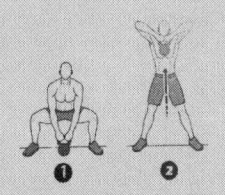

Wide-stance pull kettlebell to chin, elbows high.

1. Stand with feet wider than shoulder-width apart, toes pointed outward.
2. Hold a kettlebell with both hands, arms extended downwards.
3. Lower into a sumo squat, keeping your back straight and chest up.
4. Explosively stand up, pulling the kettlebell to your chin.
5. Keep your elbows high and out during the pull.
6. Lower the kettlebell back down and repeat the movement.

Thruster

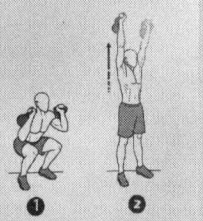

Squat to overhead press, one fluid motion with kettlebell.

1. Stand with feet shoulder-width apart, holding a kettlebell at chest level.
2. Squat down, keeping your chest up and back straight.
3. As you stand up, press the kettlebell overhead in one fluid motion.
4. Lower the kettlebell back to chest level and repeat.
5. Ensure the transition from squat to press is smooth.
6. Maintain a strong core and stable kettlebell throughout the exercise.

Torso Twist

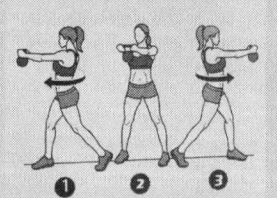

Stand, twist torso holding kettlebell across body.

1. Stand with feet shoulder-width apart, holding a kettlebell with both hands.
2. Extend your arms in front of you at chest level.
3. Twist your torso to the right, bringing the kettlebell to your side.
4. Return to the center and twist to the left.
5. Keep your hips facing forward and core engaged.
6. Repeat the twisting motion, focusing on controlled movements.

Tricep Dip

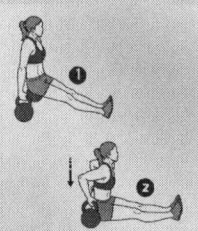

Dip using parallel bars, hold kettlebell for added weight.

1. Position yourself between parallel bars, holding a kettlebell with your feet.
2. Lower your body by bending your elbows until your upper arms are parallel to the ground.
3. Keep your elbows close to your body and your core engaged.
4. Push through your palms to extend your elbows and return to the starting position.
5. Repeat, maintaining a controlled movement throughout.
6. Focus on engaging your triceps during the dip.

Tricep Extension

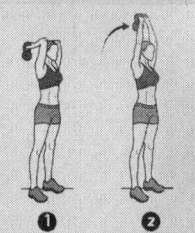

Extend arms overhead, kettlebell in hands.

1. Stand with feet shoulder-width apart, holding a kettlebell with both hands.
2. Extend your arms overhead, keeping your elbows close to your head.
3. Lower the kettlebell behind your head by bending your elbows.
4. Engage your triceps to lift the kettlebell back to the starting position.
5. Keep your core tight and avoid arching your back.
6. Repeat, ensuring controlled movements.

Turkish Get Up

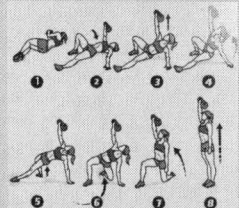

Stand from floor, kettlebell overhead, controlled motion.

1. Lie on your back with your right leg bent and right foot flat on the floor, holding a kettlebell in your right hand.
2. Extend your left arm and leg on the floor.
3. Press the kettlebell straight up, keeping your eyes on it.
4. Roll onto your left forearm, then onto your left hand.
5. Push through your right foot to lift your hips off the ground.
6. Sweep your left leg under your body to a kneeling position.
7. Stand up fully, keeping the kettlebell overhead.
8. Reverse the steps to return to the starting position.
9. Repeat on the other side.

Weighted Lunge

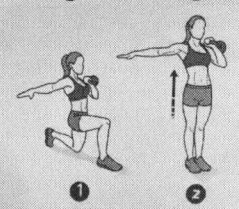

Lunge holding kettlebell to increase resistance.

1. Stand with feet shoulder-width apart, holding a kettlebell in your right hand.
2. Step forward with your left foot and lower your hips, bending both knees to 90 degrees.
3. Keep your back straight and core engaged.
4. Push through your left heel to return to the starting position.
5. Repeat on the right leg, holding the kettlebell in your left hand.
6. Focus on keeping your weight evenly distributed and maintaining balance.

Windmill

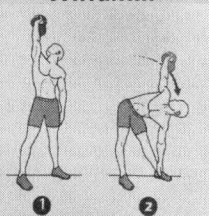

Reach toward floor, one arm overhead holding kettlebell.

1. Stand with feet shoulder-width apart, holding a kettlebell in your right hand overhead.
2. Turn your left foot out slightly and push your hips to the right.
3. Lower your torso towards the floor, keeping your right arm extended overhead.
4. Reach your left hand towards the ground, keeping your gaze on the kettlebell.
5. Engage your core to return to the starting position.
6. Repeat on the other side, switching the kettlebell to your left hand.

Wood Chop

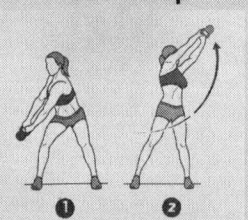

Swing kettlebell diagonally across body, squat to lift.

1. Stand with feet shoulder-width apart, holding a kettlebell with both hands.
2. Swing the kettlebell diagonally across your body, starting from your left hip.
3. Squat down slightly as you swing the kettlebell up and across to the right.
4. Engage your core and rotate your torso during the movement.
5. Reverse the motion, bringing the kettlebell back to your left hip.
6. Repeat, focusing on a smooth, controlled motion.
7. Switch sides after completing the desired number of repetitions.

Made in the USA
Columbia, SC
19 January 2025